A Dynamic Materia Medica

HELIUM

Including an Introduction to the Noble Gases

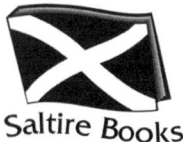
Saltire Books   *Saltire Books Limited, Glasgow, Scotland*

A Dynamic Materia Medica

HELIUM
Including an Introduction
to the Noble Gases

Jeremy Sherr

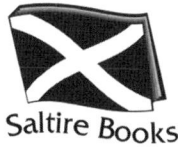 Saltire Books *Saltire Books Limited, Glasgow, Scotland*

Published by Saltire Books Ltd

18–20 Main Street, Busby, Glasgow G76 8DU, Scotland
books@saltirebooks.com   www.saltirebooks.com

Cover, Design, Layout and Text © Saltire Books Ltd 2013

 is a registered trademark

First published in 2013

Typeset by Type Study, Scarborough, UK in 9¼ on 13½ Stone Serif
Printed by Berforts Information Press Ltd, Eynsham, Oxford, UK

ISBN 978-1-908127-03-7

For Saltire
Project Development: Lee Kayne
Editorial: Steven Kayne
Designer: Phil Barker
Illustrator: Matt Canning
Indexer: Jan Worrall

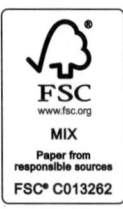

Printed on FSC® Certified Paper

CONTENTS

Dedicated to the memory of my mother,
Naomi Grace Cohen, daughter of Rabbi Moses Isaac
Cohen (MIC) and Birdie Cohen

FOREWORD BY
YAKOV MELAMED COHEN

There are seven periods in the periodic table. The end of each of these periods is punctuated by one of the noble gases which represent the fulfilment of each period's aspirations. All the preceding elements struggle through life in a constant state of lack and dissatisfaction. They are missing one or more electrons necessary to reach a state of completion, balance and harmony. This struggle represents the continuous restless motion of life. The noble gases, possessing a full house of protons and electrons, have achieved this goal. Satisfied and whole in themselves, they exist in stable, inert and isolated glory and have no need of any other element. They are monatomic: They neither bind to each other nor do they form molecules. As such, they do not participate in the messy games of chemistry and life.

The lesser elements, looking on in envy, aspire to attain this state but can only approximate it through chemical interaction and sharing of resources, namely electrons. Out of 118 elements, only seven have reached this lofty state. Like seven enlightened beings, they wander across the universe, always present but never intermingling.

If we can understand the inner nature of a noble element, we can understand the aspirations of all the preceding elements in the period, and consequently perceive what it is they are lacking. While there are many theoretical ways of reaching this understanding, the true path of knowledge in homeopathy is that of provings followed by cases. No other method can give as profound an insight into the inner nature of the elements. Provings provoke the strange, rare and peculiar; that which is unexpected and therefore not predictable by logic or theory.

This book would be impossible without the wonderful provings conducted by my friend Jeremy Sherr. Thanks to these provings, we have been able to investigate deeply this fascinating group of elements in their homeopathic and esoteric context. The editing and arrangement of provings is in itself a feat of incredibly detailed hard work, a succession of symptoms. However it is the process of analysing and ultimately synthesising the material in which the genius of these books lies, the potentising of perception.

Yaakov Melamed Cohen
January 2013

PREFACE

The elements of the periodic table are the building blocks of the universe. The noble gases are a key to understanding the periodic table. I therefore embarked on an investigation of the noble gases towards a deeper understanding of health, disease and our entire materia medica. I never imagined it would take me twenty years.

Throughout this series of books the term 'noble gases' will be used rather than 'inert gases' that is no longer considered accurate. The use of the words 'rare gases' is also inaccurate because argon forms a fairly considerable part (0.94% by volume, 1.3% by mass) of the Earth's atmosphere.

The journey began in 1993 with the proving of Neon. This was followed in 1995 by Helium and 1997 gave birth to both Krypton and Argon. My friend and colleague Silvie Gowen later proved Xenon and Radon. I reproved Xenon in 2012 and aim to follow with a proving of Radon.[i] Thus the six noble samurai are nearly complete, missing only the elusive seventh of their number, 'Element 118'.

Collectively these provings form a family of remedies, grouped together not only by their unique placement in the periodic table, but by their consequent proving symptoms. It is this family that I have set out to examine, based not on speculation, but on the correct homeopathic sequence of provings followed by perception and then by clinical cases.

The first volume in this series contains an introduction to the noble gases and an in-depth exploration of Helium, which is the leading light and gateway to all the other nobles. I aim to follow with the other nobles, and perhaps even the seventh son. Some of these remedies are more familiar to me than others. I am very well acquainted with Helium, Neon, Argon, and Krypton, while Xenon and Radon are currently less familiar. No doubt reproving and writing about them will summon more cases and further my understanding.

---

[i] At this time we are having technical difficulties in obtaining pure radon.

The ultimate volume in this series will attempt to reach some conclusions regarding the noble gases as a family and to use the knowledge gained to investigate the related rows of elements and the entire periodic table: its aspirations, limitations and clinical applications. Furthermore, I hope to venture beyond clinical concepts by using the understanding gained to take a peek into the related mysteries of our existence.

I have worked on Helium for a period of ten years, navigating unchartered territories, dwelling on it secrets during wake and dream time. Perhaps the nature of this remedy was reflected in the multitude of ideas which had difficulty manifesting into the 'real' world. Time and again I happily announced to my wife that the book was finished, only to find myself tearing it all apart and struggling with the concepts once again. The noble gas series is certainly one of the most difficult intellectual challenges I have ever faced. It has taken the best of my ability to unravel some of the codes hidden within these provings. Not so much in the lower potencies of perception, for that was straight forward, but rather the higher realms are those which provided the challenge. For while clinical application of this knowledge is the purpose of this investigation and the test of its validity, there are deeper aspects which demand exploration. Ideas have come and gone, and no doubt will continue to do so after publication. More mysteries will be uncovered in time, others will remain concealed. Mistakes will be discovered, and changes will be made. I therefore present this series as a hypothesis, my personal interpretation of these provings, a suggestion to those who have the will and talent to take it further. I appreciate any feedback, suggestions and relevant cases.

The provings of the noble gases are a true wonder, an endless voyage of discovery, both as individual remedies and as a group. One characteristic of the noble gases is that they emit light when an electric current flows through them. It is my hope that these books will supply you, my homeopathic friend, with some of the voltage needed to enlighten your homeopathic journey.

Notes

Elements beginning with a small letter represent chemical atoms, while elements beginning with a capital represent their related remedies.

Text in blue type represents proving symptoms.

All poems are by Jeremy Sherr unless otherwise indicated.

The complete proving of Helium is available online at www.dynamis.edu

ABOUT THE AUTHOR

Jeremy Sherr has practiced and taught homeopathy for 33 years. He has clinics in London, New York and Tel Aviv and is principle of 'The Dynamis School for Advanced Homoeopathic Medicine' one of the longest running post-graduate courses in the world. Jeremy has taught homeopathy throughout the USA and Europe, as well as in Canada, China, India, Israel, Mexico, Japan, Russia, South Africa, New Zealand and Australia.

He has conducted 34 classical homeopathic provings and is the author of *The Dynamics and Methodology of Homoeopathic Provings, Dynamic Materia Medica Volume I-Syphilis, Dynamic Provings Volumes I and II, and The Repertory of Mental Qualities*. He has published numerous articles on homeopathy and has conducted several research programs.

Since 2008 Jeremy has been living in Tanzania where, together with his wife Camilla, he has set up rural clinics and is working in the local hospital. They have treated over 2500 AIDS patients and have established food programs and a day care centre for children with AIDS.

ACKNOWLEDGEMENTS

I wish to thank the following people for their invaluable help in creating this book:

To Silvie Gowan for her most wonderful provings. Silvie has been a fellow traveller on the noble journey since the beginning. With her amazing ability to listen to whispers, Silvie's unique provings are a true wonder. Other than the magic, Silvie has put a tremendous amount of work into arranging and editing her provings.

To all the Norwegian provers, supervisors and editors at Dynamis School Norway 1995 and in particular Ingrid High, the proving editor.

To Sarah Hemsley and Ceridwen Edwards of Aurora Provings.

To John Morgan and Helios pharmacy for preparing the remedy

Many thanks to Vivien Freund for editing, critical evaluation and help with esoteric mathematics. Finding a great homeopathic logician in deepest Africa was a true gift. Vivien's keen mind and tenacity helped me crack some tough conundrums.

My editor Richenda Gillespie has turned this book into a professional presentation. I thank her for her excellent skills, dedication and perfectionism.

To Andreas Bjørndal for review, advice and generous sharing of resources. Andreas is a fountain of knowledge and more importantly a great synthesiser. He also took part in the Helium proving.

Thanks to Linda Johnston and Franz Vermeulen for encouraging words and for recommending Steven and Lee Kayne from Saltire publishers. That turned out to be a great decision. To the wonderful team at Saltire Books, who publish with real care.

Special thanks to my mentor Rabbi Yaakov Melamed Cohen for his wisdom and teaching.

The following people have helped with comments, editing, repertorising and cases: Christopher Beaver, Shelly Been, Lilia Dimitrova, Lukas Gold, Jacqueline Hobbs, Jacob Kiakahi, Yael Langford Z'al, Jeremy Langford, Rosie

Nightingale, Becca Preston, Tina Quirk, Camilla Sherr, Katrin Sigwart, Liz Thompson, Kåre Troelsen and Yorik Verete and to anyone I have forgotten. Thank you all!

To Brenda Brown for Figure 4.1 and to the University of Science & Philosophy for permission to use diagrams by Walter Russell.

And to my wife Camilla Malka Sherr, for whom I write.

part one

THE NOBLE GASES
AN INTRODUCTION TO THE SERIES

A BRIEF EXPLANATION OF THE PERIODIC TABLE AND THE NOBLE GASES

The noble gases provide us with a key with which to unlock the periodic table. Many homeopaths have difficulty understanding the periodic table, often due to inadequate teaching of chemistry at school. I will begin by offering a simplified explanation for those who have suffered from a poor introduction to chemistry, although expert chemists may also gain some insights from it. Even if you have a sound understanding of the periodic table, I recommend reading this introduction to help you understand the noble gases as homeopathic remedies.

While our perception of atoms and subatomic particles has advanced substantially during most of the last 100 years, the older planetary model of the atom suffices for our purposes. This solar system model was first proposed by Niels Bohr in 1913.[1] The basic idea is that an atom is made up of a core nucleus surrounded by electrons that orbit this nucleus.

To give some perspective, if a proton were the size of London's Royal Albert Hall, an electron would be a speck of dust whizzing around it at a distance of 3 kilometres. Most of matter is composed of empty space.

Thirteen billion years ago, a mere 400 million years after the Big Bang, the universe cooled down enough to allow the formation of the first two elements: hydrogen and helium. These elements form the first period of the periodic table and are the main constituents of the process we call 'sun'. In the sun, hydrogen atoms fuse into helium, a process that releases a huge amount of energy.

Hydrogen is the simplest atom in the universe. Composed of just one electron and one proton, it has the atomic number one. Protons are positively charged subatomic particles, whereas electrons are negatively charged. Protons are essentially female energy, residing in the nucleus of the atom and providing it with mass and substance, while the negatively charged and essentially male electrons whiz around the nucleus at high speed. According to quantum mechanics, an electron is both a wave and a particle that is present everywhere simultaneously due to its great speed.

A positive proton and a negative electron create an electrical balance. Most atoms also have one or more neutrons in their nuclei; however this carries no known electrical charge. Other than adding weight to the atom, a neutron has no chemical significance. The isotope of hydrogen which has one extra neutron is known as deuterium and the isotope with two extra neutrons is known as tritium. Since the first H bomb experiments in 1954, it is no longer possible to obtain pure hydrogen, as a certain amount of deuterium or heavy hydrogen is present everywhere, even locked within icebergs. The only exception is wine bottled before this date. As most of us cannot afford such wine, or would prefer to drink it rather than subjecting it to chemical analysis, all provings of hydrogen contain a proportion of its heavier isotopes.

An atom that is missing its electron is known as an ion and is positively charged. You may have heard the story of the two atoms drinking in a bar late one night. One atom asks his friend, "Why are you drinking?" The other sadly replies, "I have lost my electron." To which the first atom says, "Are you positive?"

We will now examine the periodic table from a metaphorical point of view. Hydrogen, comprised of one female proton and one male electron, represents yin and yang in perfect harmony. Lighter than air, it floats out of the atmosphere and up into space; hydrogen is the most abundant element in the universe, making up around seventy five percent of all matter. Based on its proving, homeopathic hydrogen represents unification with God on one hand and a fragmented universal soul on the other.[2]

In order to incarnate into the vast diversity of individual souls, these fragments of universal soul must separate from heaven and fuse to form a potentially gender-based soul ready to manifest in a body. The fusion of four hydrogen nuclei (proton-proton chain reaction) creates helium. Because it has two protons, helium has the atomic number 2. Though heavier than hydrogen, it is still much lighter than air and represents an individual soul. Like a helium-filled balloon, the disembodied soul floats skywards unless anchored to an earthly body.

Helium is the first noble gas, with a complete outer shell of electrons. Each noble gas affords us insight into the elements preceding it in the periodic table, their desires and aspirations. Hydrogen is the first atom to originate from the undivided singularity, the primary unit which contains the whole universe within. Its deepest desire therefore is to be reabsorbed back into the whole. If it cannot move back into this state of universal oneness, it must move forward towards becoming an undivided and complete soul: Helium.

Helium has a full house of subatomic particles. Two protons reside in the nucleus, and two electrons orbit this nucleus in an outer shell. This shell is physically full, meaning it has no room for any additional electrons, just as a fertilised egg will not admit a second sperm through its outer membrane. As chemical reactions occur through the sharing of electrons, helium is unable to interact chemically.

We can compare Helium to an immature young person living alone a small one room apartment. He does not go out much and needs no interaction with the outside world. The external world seems strange, messy and scary and he would rather remain indoors locked in his own thoughts.

Eventually, as is the world's way, he meets a nice young lady and falls in love. After the stable and fulfilled state of helium, nature rolls on into destabilised complexity. And so a second period must begin. Imagine a typist finishing a sentence. The full stop or period at the end of the sentence is the noble gas, after which we press the 'enter' key and move down to the next row, arriving at lithium.

Lithium, the third element of the periodic table, possesses three protons electrically balanced by three electrons. There is no room in the first shell of the hydrogen and helium series to add an extra electron. Therefore another shell must be formed to hold this third electron, which moves into an outer orbit where it circles at a greater distance from the nucleus. As we have moved from gases to the first solid, this process is akin to the soul acquiring a body. Lithium literally means stone, the most basic physical substance on earth, a weight that ties the soul to the ground.

Lithium therefore comprises a nucleus with three protons: two electrons in the first shell and a lonely single electron in the outer shell. Let us return to our couple in love. She is now pregnant and the one-bedroom apartment is no longer large enough to house them. They have to move into a larger two-bedroom apartment where they can prepare for the baby. But as she grows larger with each month, this apartment will quickly fill with the couples things.

After lithium, beryllium is created with four protons and four electrons: two in the inner shell and two in the outer shell. And so we proceed, filling the second shell with more and more electrons (and the nucleus with more protons), forming boron, carbon, nitrogen, oxygen, and fluorine.

By the end of the second period of the periodic table, we have all the constituents necessary for organic life. Carbon, representing a C-shaped uterus, is ready to receive a hydrogen soul. Nitrogen nourishes the foetus through the placenta, and oxygen suffuses it with the breath of life. Only after the formation of oxygen in the second period can water appear. Water, two hydrogen soul fragments bonded by oxygen, is the basis of all life. *hydro-gen* gets its name from the part it plays in the formation of water. It is interesting to note that as the lightest and most explosive of elements, Rudolf Steiner preferred to call it *pyrogen* or fire element. Water is therefore a combination of fire and air, united and transformed into the secret of life. And out of these overflowing waters, neon is born.

The second period's gestation reaches its completion in neon. Nine months and nine elements have passed from the helium conception to neon's birth. Now the waters break and new life (néon is the Greek word for new) is born. Neon has ten protons in the nucleus and ten electrons revolving around this nucleus: two electrons fill the inner shell and eight fill the outer shell. Mum and Dad in one room and eight children in the second room results in a full house. They live in their two bedroom apartment as a complete and happy family, a state of bliss. They do not go out much and need no interaction with the outside world. The second shell is now complete and it is time to move into the next period. In our analogy more children are born and the family must move into a larger house with an extra bedroom (or shell).

The first element in the third period is sodium (or *natrium* in Latin). It contains eleven protons in its nucleus and eleven orbiting electrons: two in the inner shell, eight in the second shell and one in the new third shell. Natrium is similar to lithium and hydrogen; they all contain one electron in their outer shell and thus share similar chemical properties, as do the first elements of each of the remaining periods: potassium, rubidium, caesium and francium. All these elements are highly reactive, displaying an inherent lack of stability.

It is the number of electrons in the outer shell that gives an element its chemical properties, so the cycle of similar elements is repeated in every new period. As the periodic table spirals downwards, elements with the same number of electrons in the outer shell share similar characteristics which repeat themselves, hence the name *period* (a cycle of time marked by the recurrence of some phenomenon or a recurring process). This is why we place similar elements under one another in vertical columns called groups.

In another analogy, we could say that elements within a group or column that possess similar characteristics represent a family (mother, daughter and granddaughter), while elements within a period or rows are like neighbours living in the same street. They come from the same social stratum, but they do not share similar genetic characteristics as members of a family would. Figure I.1 illustrates the differences between a period and a group.

The third period fills up in a similar way to the second. After neon the couple gives birth to a sodium child. After sodium, magnesium arrives with twelve protons and twelve electrons, then aluminium, silicon and so on, until the fulfilment of the period is reached in argon. Argon is element number 18; it has two electrons in its inner shell, eight in the second and eight more in its third shell. The oldest child is now eighteen years old and in his prime. End of sentence, full stop, press return. Once again the noble gas has accomplished the whole period's aspirations as youth matures into a young adult, ready for life and procreation. In the next period, period number four, it is time to buy a few houses for the grandchildren. The family has now evolved into a tribe or village. In a village people share skills and resources and so professions evolve: You do my carpentry and I'll do your plumbing.

The fourth shell, lying further from the nucleus, has a larger orbit and can hold eighteen electrons rather than the maximum eight as in the second and third periods. The element with atomic number 36, krypton, completes this period with a full house of 18 electrons in its outer shell. Krypton represents the mature professional, thus completing the cycle of work.

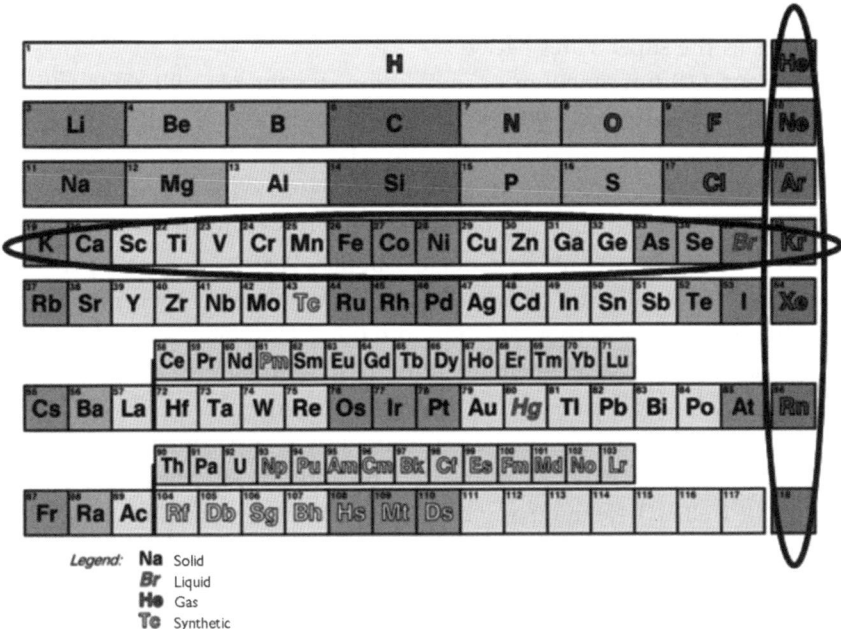

Figure I.1 *Periodic table of the elements (highlighting column 8 and row 4)*

In the fifth period, great-grandchildren are born and villages amalgamate into cities. Distances grow and transport, communication and cash become the means of transaction. Rather than swapping professional skills, money becomes the means of exchange (*argent*/money, *argentum*/silver). The remedy Argentum Metallicum affects nerve sheaths and hence long-distance neural communication in the body. This period finds its completion in xenon, which has 54 electrons in total and a full quota of 18 electrons in its outer shell.[i] Xenon completes the period of higher professional achievement though a vocation such as doctor, banker, scientist, musician, artist or priest.

The final two periods, periods six and seven, have even larger outer orbits. Both of these periods are completed by noble gases with a full quote of 32 electrons in their fullest shells. Once again we have a full house. In the sixth period cities have bonded together to form kingdoms, countries and corporations in which kings, CEOs and rulers hold unbounded sway. Power supersedes money as the dominant factor.

The seventh period is the radioactive one. The elements of this final period are so large and unstable that they emit particles and waves in the form of radiation. In our analogy countries have now amalgamated to super-states, giant and unstable unions composed of many smaller countries. The USSR, USA, China, India and the European common market are examples of these super states, where peripheral countries lie far from the control of central governments and are thus emitted like radioactive particles as the super-states decay.

Element 118 (ununoctium or uuo) completes the periodic table with a full shell of 32 electrons. This element is so unstable that it does not exist naturally on earth, though erroneous claims of its production were published in 1998, 2002 and 2005. The most recent claim was made on the 16 October 2006, the same day I began writing this book. In the same week North Korea detonated its first nuclear bomb. Five years later Japan has gone through the disaster of Fukushima, leaving a boiling pot on the verge of spilling huge amounts of radiation into our atmosphere. As element 118 is the last radioactive element, it only exists naturally in conditions of extreme heat and pressure such as those found in supernovas. I have named it luciferium after Lucifer, the bearer of light, who according to one myth was said to be the archangel closest to God and was later banished to the depths of Hell.[3] There are many connotations of the name Lucifer. In the old testament he is referred to as the 'morning star'.[4] One can speculate

---

[i] This is not strictly true as xenon has the complete quota of 18 electrons in its 4th rather than 5th shell, but the layout of shell configuration in atoms is beyond the scope of this book.

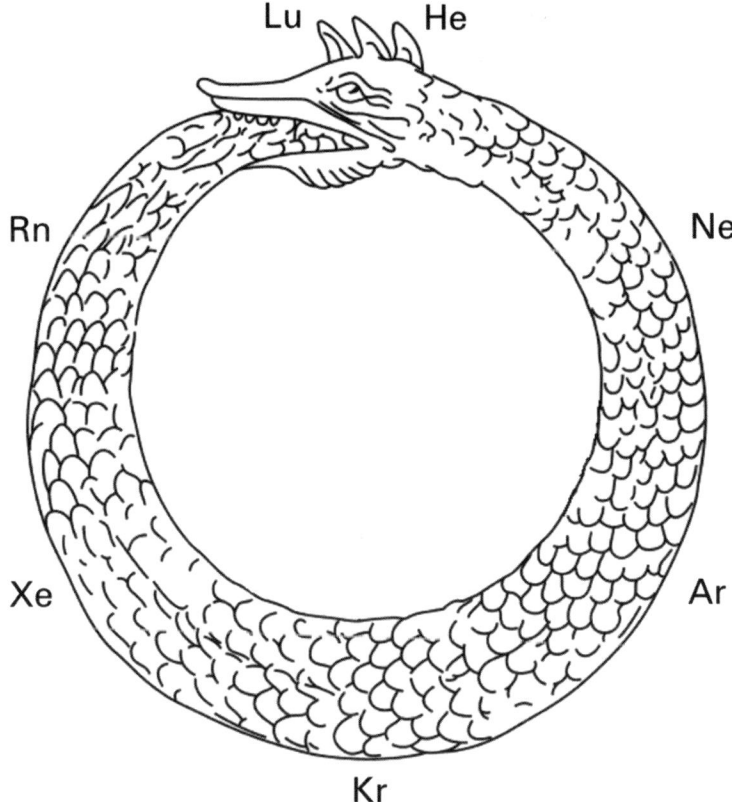

Figure I.2 *The ouroboros or serpent eating its own tail*

that its discovery will complete the process of creation and represent the end (or new beginning) of life on earth as we know it.

The radioactive elements in the seventh period release alpha, beta and gamma radiation. Alpha radiation is in fact an ejected helium nucleus. Therefore there is a relationship between the seventh radioactive period and the first period, a completion of the spiral where the snake bites its own tail (see Figure I.2).

The radioactive period is associated with the deepest layers of nature, body and culture: bone marrow, cell nuclei, genes, genetics, generations, ancestry, territory, immunity, underground, roots, collective and subconscious mind, fungi, the internet, cancer and AIDS. It is also related to powers that are able to influence and control kingdoms in a veiled manner from behind the scenes: shamans, wizards, magicians, jesters and jokers such as Rasputin, and giant commercial networks like pharmaceutical companies that can manipulate governments to create enormous wealth and power.

The development of the periodic table also marks the evolution of time and space. While hydrogen and helium exist in deep space since the beginnings of the universe, the elements of the second period were born of exploding stars and supernovas billions of years ago. Being heavier, they may be trapped in earth's atmosphere. Sulphur, alumina, magnesium and other elements of the third period formed the crust of our cooling planet. Three thousand years ago we began mining for iron, silver and gold, digging ever deeper into the earth's layers. Today we mimic the pressure and heat which furnace the centre of our planet to create radioactive elements that will decay in less than a millisecond.

This concludes our introduction to the periodic table of elements, a wonderful spiral representing the descent and development of nature and humankind. There is some interesting numerology attached to the periodic table. One such example of the mathematical beauty and logic of its numbers is illustrated in Figure I.3 below.

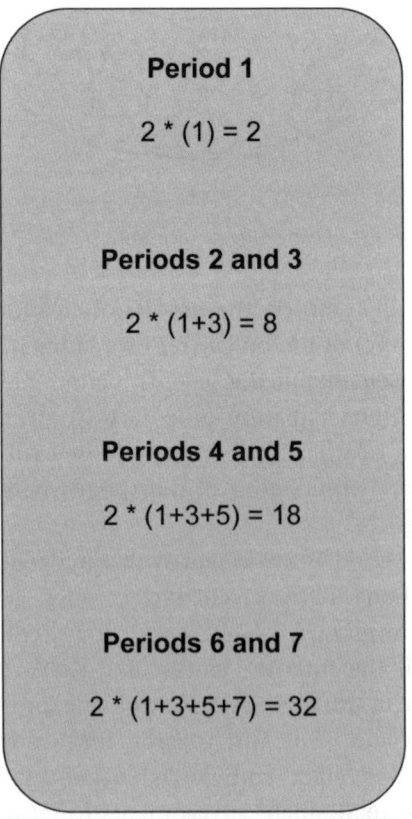

Period 1

$2 * (1) = 2$

Periods 2 and 3

$2 * (1+3) = 8$

Periods 4 and 5

$2 * (1+3+5) = 18$

Periods 6 and 7

$2 * (1+3+5+7) = 32$

Figure I.3 Formulae for the number of electrons in the outer shell

One of the most interesting numerological descriptions I have come across lies in the following diagram, designed by my friend Andreas N. Bjørndal. This diagram demonstrates the basic numerology based on quantum physics and shows a beautiful symmetry between columns and rows. It is based on the configuration of the shells or orbitals of each element. Thus the knowledge reflected in this diagram takes us one degree further in the path of understanding the periodic table. Andreas has promised to explore this diagram more fully in one of the following books of this series.

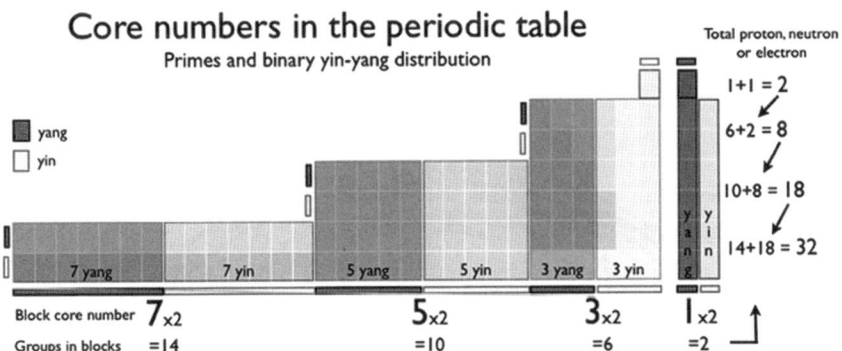

Figure I.4 *Andreas Bjørndal's periodic table*
Reproduced with kind permission of the author

Chemical interactions

The noble gases are also known as inert gases as they have no need to mix with the other elements. They exist in perfect and glorious isolation. All other elements strive to be as complete and fulfilled as the noble gases. The only way they can achieve this is by sharing their electrons.

Take the case of two teenagers: young Mr Natrium and the attractive Miss Chlorine. They meet on the beach one day and immediately fall in love. He has one extra electron in his outer shell. To emulate the noble state of a full outer shell he can either retreat to the infantile neon or move forward towards his idol, the youthful argon of Neverland. With seven electrons in her outer shell Miss Chlorine needs only one more electron to reach the argon fairytale marriage. If he can introduce his electron into her, the union will be fruitful and complete. After losing his electron Mr Natrium becomes a positively charged ion Na+, and after gaining his electron Miss Chlorine becomes the negatively charged ion Cl−. They are now bonded to each other through electrical attraction, an ionic bond.

Naïvely believing that they are the perfect match, the two ions hold their wedding on the beach. They become the family Natrium Muriaticum or common salt. Henceforth they will live happily ever after in virtual simulation of their noble heroes. That is unless their love goes into dissolution. When the solid salt crystal dissolves in water, the ions are released into the solution, where they become attached to the polar charged water molecules. Natrium and sodium ions are now separated from each other by seas of grief. He leaves his heart with her while she carries his extra electron child. The chemical formula of love disappointment looks like this:

$$NaCl(s) + H2O(l) \rightarrow H2O(l) + Na+(aq) + Cl-(aq)$$

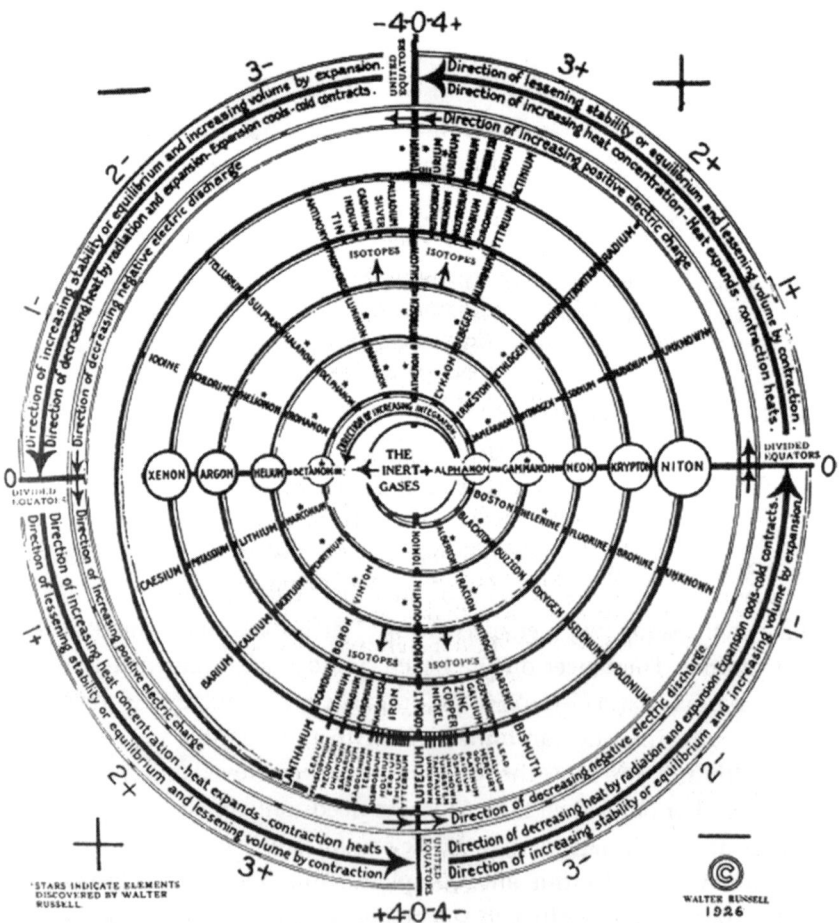

Figure I.5 *The noble gases are in the centre*

Diagram of the periodic table by Walter Russell, courtesy of the University of Science & Philosophy

The complete octet can also be achieved by a co-valent bond. An example is co-valent bonding with carbon. With four electros in its outer shell carbon has what is termed a valence of four. The carbon atom can thus combine with four chlorine atoms to give each a stable group of eight and at the same time giving the carbon atom a stable group of eight; thus we have carbon tetrachloride. Happy families.

All chemical bonds, from those found in simple chemical combinations to those in giant organic molecules, are based on this attempt to emulate noble stability. Water or H_20 shares 10 protons and electrons, the same number as the noble neon, a similarity that is clearly reflected in the watery proving of Neon. What we cannot achieve alone can be achieved through sharing. One of the tasks of proving noble gas remedies is to enquire whether possessing solitary perfection (as a noble gas) is comparable or even preferable to the simulated wholeness achieved by sharing (as chemical compounds). In other words, how does a supposedly perfect individual compare to a loving group of mortals that have learnt to combine their assets.

Alternative periodic tables

There are hundreds of different diagrams depicting the periodic table. Most place a noble gas at the end of each period. Occasionally, the noble gases are depicted centrally (see Figure I.5). Arguably the most realistic depiction of the periodic table shows it in a spiral shape (as illustrated in Figure I.6), where each noble gas is placed opposite the central element of its period.

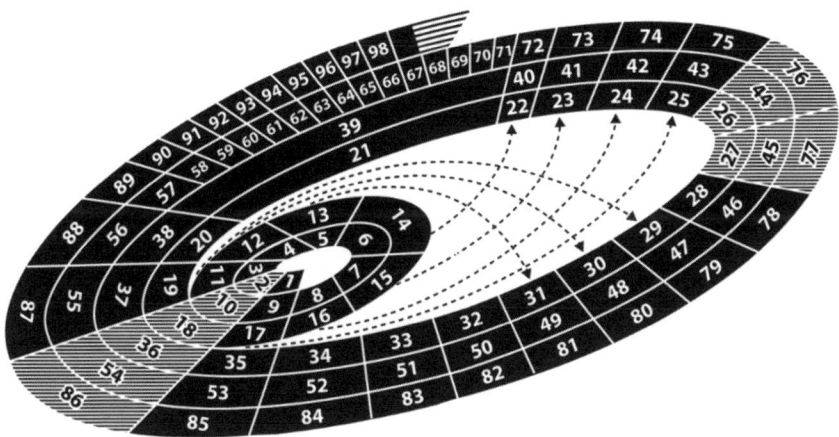

Figure I.6 *The elements arranged in order of their mass on the periodic table, illustrating the noble gases in the centre*

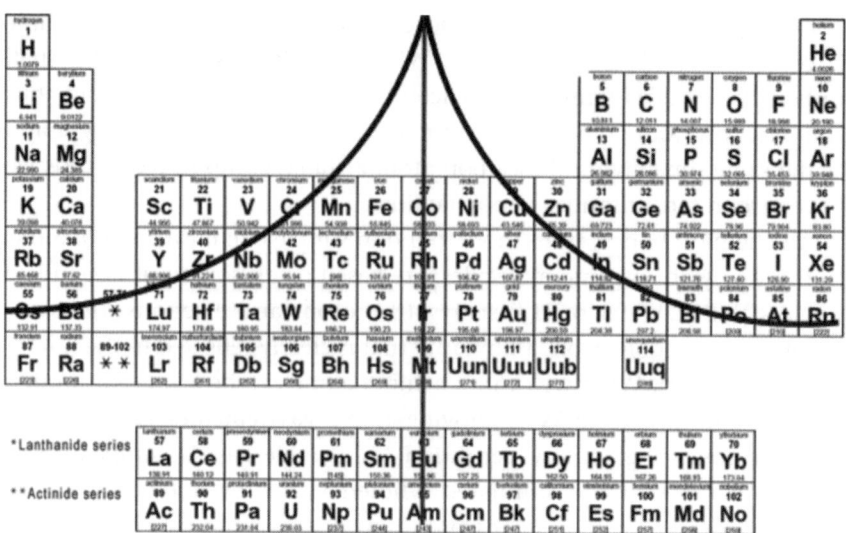

Figure I.7 *Periodic table of the elements showing the apex in the centre*

Placing the noble at the centre of each period reminds us that they belong as much to the preceding period as to the following one. Try taking a sheet of paper with the periodic table printed on it and twisting it into a spiral. In this spiral neon is directly opposite carbon and radon is opposite

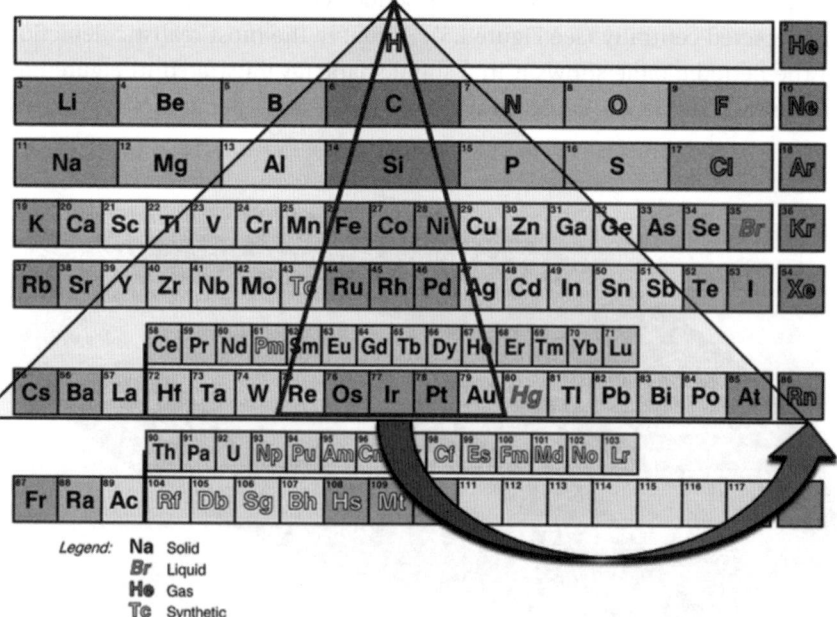

Legend: **Na** Solid
Br Liquid
He Gas
Tc Synthetic

Figure I.8 *Dynamis School periodic table showing the central line and wrap-around to corresponding noble gases*

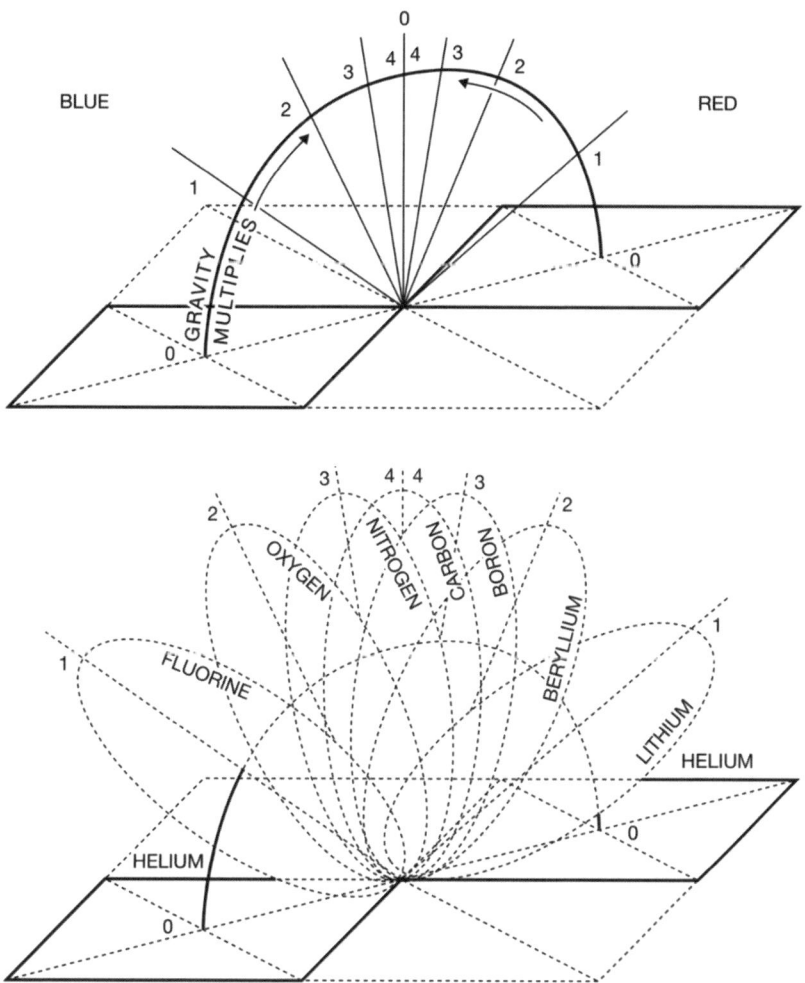

Figure I.9 *Diagram of the periodic table by Walter Russell*
Courtesy of the University of Science & Philosophy

elements 75, 76 and 77 (rhenium, osmium and iridium). The central elements carbon, silicon, cobalt, rhodium and iridium and their immediate neighbours represent the zeniths of each respective period.

The standard depiction of the periodic table shown in Figure I.7, however, not the most accurate representation, because it has been artificially stretched for convenience to form a rectangular box. Carbon is not only the mother of silicon, it is the four-armed, diamond-wedding, great-grandmother of many central elements (as can be seen in the proving of Adamas).[5] Figure I.8 shows carbon and silica in the middle and opposite to the noble gasses.

The central elements represent the very peak of material, emotional, professional and spiritual success, achievement and attainment. All the elements leading up to these central elements are upwardly mobile, while those following them are falling into failure.

At the opposite pole of the spiral to each central high-flier are the noble, enlightened ones. This idea is well represented in the diagrams from Walter Russell (Figures I.5 and I.9), where the central element carbon is depicted standing vertically while the inert gases are horizontal.

Contrasting a noble gas with the central element of its period is analogous to contrasting the Buddha with Genghis Khan or Lao Tzu with Steve Jobs: Enlightenment and serenity versus the precarious peak of success.

Clinical-based essences and speculative materia medica

Several contemporary homeopaths have arrived at remedy pictures of the noble gases based on speculative materia medica and clinical experiments. No doubt these pictures have helped many cases. In our modern age there is some place for the expansion of materia medica based on families, generalisations and clinical cases. We should not however imagine that these remedy pictures are entirely accurate or cover the whole totality. All too often they represent a one dimensional picture of the remedy. While unproven essences do afford initial insights, it should be remembered that these are shortcuts. In the long run such shortcuts may inhibit the unfolding of a fuller and broader totality.

For example, while the proposition of noble gases as remedies for autism has helped some patients, in my experiences it has hindered broader applications of these remedies. Only a small percentage of autistic cases respond to noble gases and the noble gases are indicated for many conditions besides autism. Too often I have seen young homeopaths adopting the suggestion of a quick essence as the be all and end all of a remedy. The problem is that while these suggestions may be true, they sell the whole truth short. This is not the path of classical homeopathy.

It is easy to create a cycle of "what we know is what we get". As long as one prescribes on the basis of speculative materia medica, these prescriptions will include only those limited aspects of the remedy that have been hypothesised upon, thus perpetuating and confirming these assumptions exclusively. If, for example, one predicts that Krypton is a remedy for having a break from work, these are the cases one will always see, thus missing the many other facets of Krypton such as time-keeping, riddle-solving, hieroglyphs, Tibetan Buddhism, stars, sky burials, birds and aliens, as well as the many peculiarities, generals, particulars, sensations, modalities, extensions and concomitants.

While speculation and quick essences may speed us along the path of clinical achievement, they are often very simplistic. It is vital to create a solid, dependable long term foundation of materia medica. In the age of fast food it is up to us homeopaths to bake wholesome holistic meals. Conducting, editing and collating provings is a long and tedious labour that does not fit our fast-paced world, but classical homeopathic provings are and will forever be our noble path of truth. Provings are the foundations on which the science, art and magic of our profession are based. They provide us with the detailed indications upon which we can practice, confirm or rule out symptoms. Provers chant the melody and rhythm of the remedy, the inner voice which we can match to the simple language of the patient. They present a window to the secrets of the universe and conjure up strange, rare and peculiar symptoms, which can never be predicted by logical systems of thought.[i]

> There is, therefore, no other possible way in which the peculiar effects of medicines on the health of individuals can be accurately ascertained – there is no sure, no more natural way of accomplishing this object, than to administer the several medicines experimentally, in moderate doses, to healthy persons, in order to ascertain what changes, symptoms and signs of their influence each individually produces on the health of the body and of the mind.[6]

While provings provide an accurate base, they can be extremely difficult to understand. Raw provings should be untangled and distilled by perceiving the pattern that binds symptoms into one comprehensive totality. That is the purpose of this book.

My questions regarding the noble gases

In analysing the provings of the noble gases, I have endeavoured to answer some of the questions that have intrigued me regarding these remedies as analogies to the human condition:

- Is the achievement of noble perfection an asset or a liability?
- Does the inertness of the noble gases result in a state of isolation and loneliness?

---

[i] See also Hahnemann's *Organon* footnotes to §6, §54 and §110.[6]

- Do these remedies manifest a state of pathological perfectionism?
- Do they portray an image that is diametrically opposite to that of noble completion, in other words a sense of dissatisfaction? And if this is the case, what flavour does this dissatisfaction possess?
- How does the noble state relate to the preceding elements and to those that follow?
- What is the lesson each noble learns, and what is its question to the next period?

One physical property of the noble gases is their curious tendency to glow and emit light when charged with electricity. Thus we have artificial lights that use helium, neon, argon (the common light bulb), krypton (torches, laser beams, car headlights) and xenon (lighthouses, fluorescent bulbs, torches, laser beams, car headlights). Like the light-bearing luciferium, all noble gases are potential emitters of light. We could speculate that these gases are inert or even lifeless due to their perfect stasis, but once galvanised with electricity, they give off an enlightened glow. What would be the nature of this electric current in the provings and how would it affect the remedy picture?

One other point arises when comparing 'ordinary' elements to their associated noble gas. In seeking noble perfection, should ordinary elements strive forward to the next noble level or back toward the preceding one? Do they aspire to acquire more protons and electrons to achieve completion or do they try and lose these subatomic particles and return to the previous noble gas? By sharing its electron with chlorine, does sodium aspire to build its quota of electrons towards argon? Should it simply lose its electron and transform back to neon as a shorter path to perfection? To look at the question in a somewhat different light: Do we gain happiness and completion by acquiring more of life's treasures or by relinquishing some of them, as many philosophies advocate?

While the elements appear to strive forwards, we may find them longing for the preceding state. For instance, Hydrogen seems to yearn to return to God (period zero), while Helium desires to return to God and yet it must move forward into organic life (period two). Natrium may long to return to the mother (in the second period), yet also strives towards the youthful romance of Argon. The work-oriented, serious-minded Kali may seek Krypton's perfect work cycle or he may yearn for the days of his carefree youth (in the third period). Luciferium, element 118, concludes the periodic table and yet recycles back to the first period by emitting helium nuclei, reflecting its proximity to God's creation as well as the ultimate destruction of the world. The periodic table is a helix that revolves forward

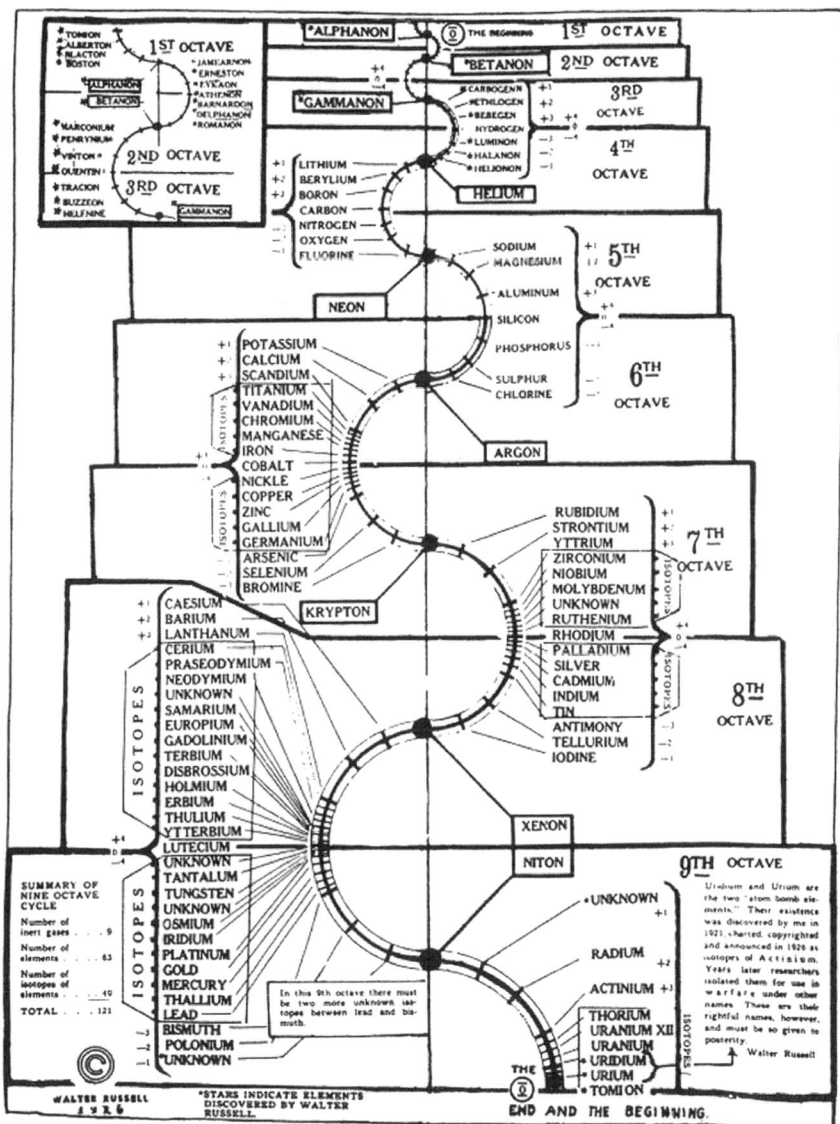

Figure I.10 *Diagram of the peridodic table by Walter Russell*
Courtesy of the University of Science & Philosophy

and backwards, ascending and descending the ladder of creation, as can be seen in Figure I.10.

Esoteric speculations on the number seven

As there are seven periods and seven noble gases, it invites a comparison with other systems based on the number seven. This was one of the a priori speculations I had in mind before embarking on the analysis of the provings and it is up to the reader to assess how well my suppositions are verified in practice. I have been more than impressed by the ultimate validity of some of these theories. The various relationships will be elaborated in association with each remedy, and the following serves only as an introduction.

The seven chakras

One system based on the number seven is the chakra system in which each chakra corresponds to one of the endocrinal glands (see Figure I.11).

It would seem logical that helium represents the crown chakra (pineal gland), neon the brow chakra (pituitary gland), argon the throat chakra (thyroid), krypton the heart chakra (thymus), xenon the solar plexus (pancreas), radon the sexual chakra (adrenal glands) and luciferium the root chakra (gonads). These speculations have been borne out nicely in the provings.

There are various versions regarding whether the root chakra is associated with the adrenals or with the gonads. In my opinion the gonads, rather than representing sexuality, represent the continuity of the generations (genes, genetics, DNA) and therefore correspond to the root chakra. The corresponding radioactive period is closely associated with genes and the

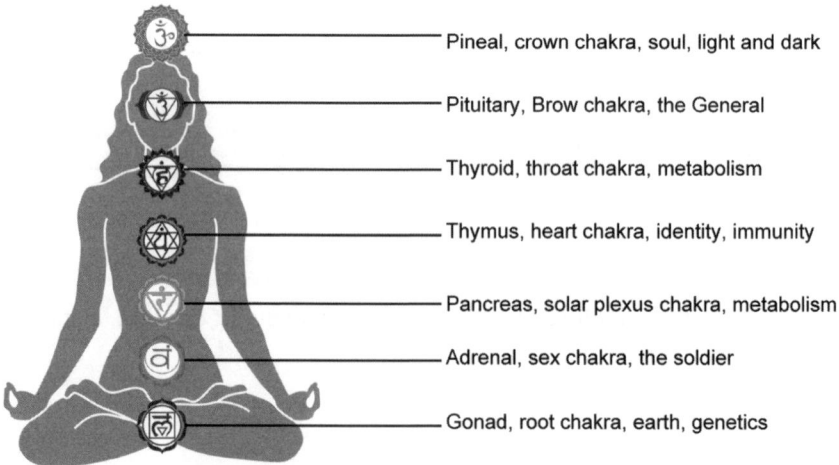

Figure I.11 *The seven chakras*

nuclei of cells and atoms, as well as with bone marrow: the deepest layers of the body. The adrenals are more akin to raw sexuality, the drive and power behind reproduction, and as such are related to the sixth period.

The seven scale octave and colours of the rainbow

Another system based on the number seven is the notes of the western musical octave comprising the notes: C, do / D, re / E, mi / F, fa / G, so / A, la / B, ti

We can compare these notes to the seven noble gases starting with helium as note B. Although there are different opinions about the musical notations, frequencies, and colours associated with the chakras, I have included the most common opinion, this according to Rodney Collins, a student of Gurdjief and Ouspensky and originator of the 'law of octaves'.[7] It should however be noted that Walter Russell compared the octave notes to each the eight elements of the second period of the periodic table.

Another conceivable analogy can be made between the noble gases and the seven colours of the rainbow. In this case helium would relate to violet whereas luciferium would relate to red.[8,9]

I have summed the correspondences up in Table I.1:

TABLE I.1   Table of correspondences with noble gases

Noble gas	Chakra	Gland	Colour	Musical note
Helium	Crown	Pineal	Violet	B, ti
Neon	Brow	Pituitary	Indigo	A, la
Argon	Throat	Thyroid	Blue	G, so
Krypton	Heart	Thymus	Green	F, fa
Xenon	Solar Plexus	Pancreas	Yellow	E, mi
Radon	Sexual	Adrenal	Orange	D, re
Luceferium	Root – Sacral	Gonad	Red	C, do

The seven stages of the alchemical process

The Hermetic tradition presents seven stages of the alchemical process, which is both chemical and spiritual. The alchemists believed there was a formula to alchemical transmutation which could be experienced if these seven operations or stages were followed. These are calcination, dissolution, separation, conjunction, fermentation, distillation and coagulation. We will examine their relevance in relation to each noble gas.

The seven days of creation in the Bible

The Bible begins with the story of the seven days of creation:

> In the beginning, God created the heavens and the earth.
> The earth was without form and void, and darkness was over the face of the deep.
> And the Spirit of God was hovering over the face of the waters.
> And God said, "Let there be light," and there was light.
> And God saw that the light was good.
> And God separated the light from the darkness.
> God called the light Day, and the darkness he called Night.
> And there was evening and there was morning, the first day.

While meditating on the noble gases, it occurred to me that there might be some correspondence between these gases and the biblical account of creation. I was extremely surprised to find how accurately this theory was borne out in the provings. According to this notion Helium would relate to the first day, Neon to the second and so on until Luciferium, which would relate to the Sabbath. I will return to this theme in each proving and in the concluding volume on the noble gases. This correspondence will afford us a two way insight, both into the noble gasses and into the biblical story. Figure I.12 shows the noble gases as they relate to the days of creation.

The seven states of process

Arthur Middleton Young (1905–1995) was an American inventor, helicopter pioneer, cosmologist, philosopher, astrologer and author. He developed the theory of process. Arthur Young explained that the evolution of Universe occurs in seven discrete states of process:[10]

- Light
- Articles
- Atoms
- Molecules
- Plants
- Animals
- Humans

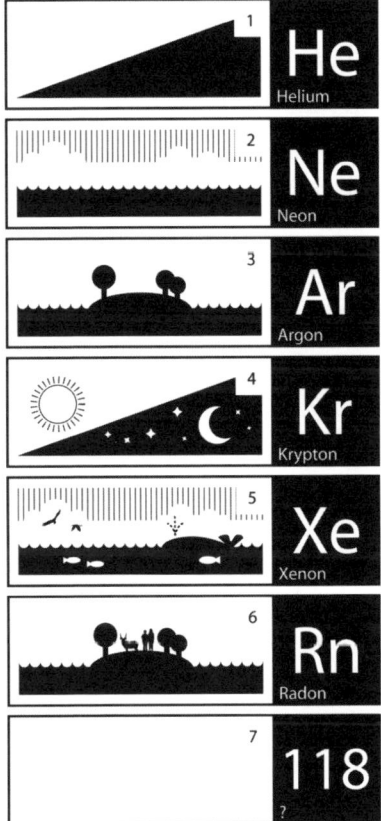

Figure I.12 The first six noble gases relating to the six days of creation

In the evolution of the seven stages of process in Universe we see that each stage develops a new power, a power that is characteristic of its stage and that differentiates it from the other stages.

And these powers are cumulative; each stage of process retains the powers developed in the previous stages. As the following diagram illustrates (see Figure I.13) there is a V shaped process in which the first four levels lose freedom by increments, while the following three gain a more controlled freedom. It remains to be seen if this model fits the developmental process of the seven periods.

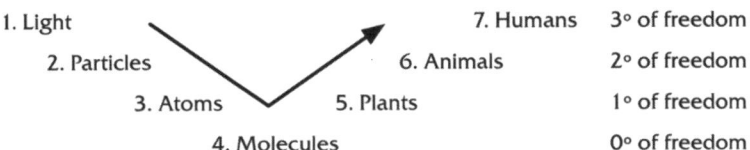

1. Light   7. Humans   3º of freedom
   2. Particles   6. Animals   2º of freedom
      3. Atoms   5. Plants   1º of freedom
         4. Molecules   0º of freedom

Figure I.13 The Arc of Process

A few more sevens

It should also be noted the there are seven orifices in the head and seven major parts of the body. Ancient cultures identified seven planets and their corresponding noble metals, these were:

Sun – Gold, Moon – Silver, Mercury – Quicksilver, Venus – Copper, Mars – Iron, Jupiter – Tin, Saturn – Lead.

So far I have not managed to find any correspondence between the series of these metals and planets and the periodic table sequence.

The Cabbala

The Cabbala talks of the seven halls or palaces (*hekhalot*), in the myth of the Merkabah (The Holy Chariot). The Merkabah homilies consisted of detailed descriptions of multiple layered heavens, seven in number, guarded over by angels, and encircled by flames and lightning. The highest heaven contains seven palaces and in the innermost palace resides a supreme divine image (God's Glory or an angelic image) seated on a throne, surrounded by awesome hosts who sing God's praise.

The seven whammies

Throughout my clinical work in homeopathy, I have observed patients aspiring and striving towards satisfaction and completion in seven different aspects of life: spirituality, intellect, relationships, occupation, society, sex/wealth/power and the home/territory. Most patients have achieved satisfaction in one or more of these, but few achieve satisfaction on all seven levels.

I have associated each of these fields of aspiration with one of the periods, with its completion manifesting as the noble gas. The reasons for these associations will be elaborated upon with each noble gas:

- Helium: Spiritual
- Neon: Structure-Intellect
- Argon: Relationships
- Krypton: Occupation
- Xenon: Self-realisation/friends
- Radon: Sex-Wealth-power
- Luciferium: Home-territory-heritage

It is interesting to note the pairs of complementary opposites working from up-down and down-up:

- Spiritual-home (periods 1 and 7)
- Structure-wealth (periods 2 and 6)
- Relationships to Self, friends and family (periods 3 and 5)
- And right in the middle: Occupation, man's mission (period 4). For a correspondence between these couplets and the chakra system (see Figure I.14).

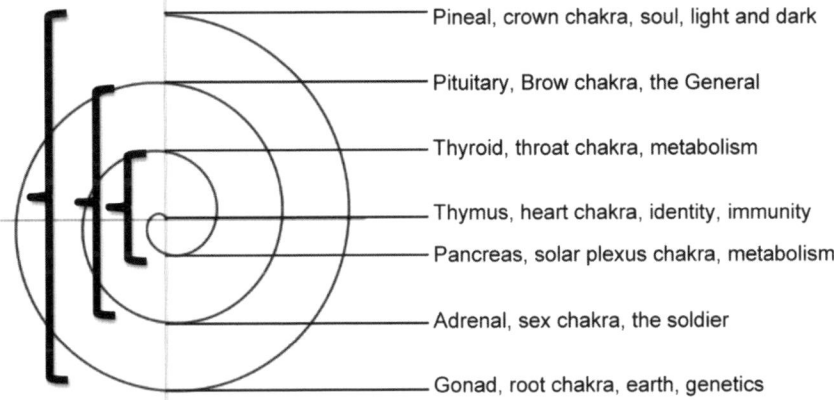

Pineal, crown chakra, soul, light and dark

Pituitary, Brow chakra, the General

Thyroid, throat chakra, metabolism

Thymus, heart chakra, identity, immunity

Pancreas, solar plexus chakra, metabolism

Adrenal, sex chakra, the soldier

Gonad, root chakra, earth, genetics

Figure I.14 The seven chakras with corresponding endocrine glands and functions

While the attainment of one or more of these goals does bring about satisfaction, it is interesting to note that this does not necessarily lead to happiness. Perhaps this is one of the many lessons that can be learned from the noble gases.

Furthermore, it is only by attaining the combined and harmonious aspirations of all the periods: spirituality, intellect, relationship, profession, family, wealth and home, representing the totality of man's desires, that we can achieve ultimate wholeness. It seems that the seven noble samurai may have to share after all.

One night, while drinking a beer with my then 19 year-old daughter, I told her about the seven whammies. While she appreciated the theory, she answered, "Dad, I have seven different whammies." These were sleep, smoking, sex, showers, coffee, talking and music.

I knew I had been outsmarted.

But seeing as it was by my own daughter, it made me more than happy.

Final questions

The final questions that arise are these:

- Can the noble gases achieve perfection in their inert state or does it require the electricity of life to galvanise them into enlightenment?
- Can the total experience of life be achieved without venturing into the imperfect and contaminated neediness of earthly existence? Do we need to experience the challenges faced by the "lesser" elements?
- Does the flawlessness of each individual noble gas result in the perfect fulfilment of health, or do they need to achieve this fulfilment as a group of seven?
- Does achieving completion of the seven whammies bring about happiness or merely inert perfection?
- Which of the various models based on the number seven that we have listed will fit the evolution of the periodic table, and how will that further our understanding?

It is my hope that by studying the noble gas provings we can begin to understand our aspirations and limitations as human beings, so that together, we can evolve towards the higher purpose of our existence.

The Periodic shuffle

Delivering the promise
Iridium Child of Heaven
radiates angelic light,
which prisms into seven.

She leaves half-sister Platina
confined by division
to step into stepmother's house
with laughter and derision.

While old King Aurum sadly
grasps his golden crown,
and yearns for unattainable
on the long climb down,
commanding General Mercury,
messenger on wings,
"Repulse the enemy without,
cause tyranny within."

Force poor Thallium's dissident
to gross emaciation,
with torture and electric shocks,
deep degeneration.

While Plumbum the dull fugitive
evades assassination,
by fleeing from lead bullets and
escaping toxication.

And down the shelter Bismuth
feeling very threatened,
clings tightly to his mummy
and begs for her protection
from the shadow of his
nuclear neighbour,
deep under the ground,
stalking shades of dead at night,
hunting with his hound.

So take me back, Iridium
seven times eleven,
colour Plumbum's heavy grey
with rainbows from the heaven,
kiss poor Thallium's balding head,
turn Mercury to mild,
heal Platina's division,
cuddle Bismuth's child,

Raise King Aurum's
self esteem,
turn him upside down,
to realise that
in his heart
lies the real crown.

For every kingdom's
bound to fall
through life's degeneration,
the only peace
lies in the noble
moment of mutation.

From sunny Helium's
Neon sky
to Argon's Peter Pan
From Krypton stars
and Xenon beasts
to Radon's upright man,
and all the way
to Luciferium,
deep beneath the ground,
between the breath
of night and day
a shaft of truth is found.

Never changing, ever still,
pivot of true life,
until the moment comes to start
the periodic slide.
A sharp electric current
turns on the noble light,
illuminating dark desires,
stillness into strife.

Carbon mother
in her taxi
riding up the mound,
four arms clutching
her organics,
one for every child:
Hydrogen, Nitrogen
Oxygen, big C,
it's relatives like Adamas
who make it clear to see:
the motto for us carbons is,
It's all to do with me,
no matter your significance,
but how you are perceived.

Then all the way
up to Iridium
starts the weary climb;
if only we would realise
we're climbing upside down
and driving grimly forward
via the mirror in reverse,
with each electron we acquire
comes a blessed curse.
So like a moth
into a flame
our proton takes a dive,
the mirror that we're living through
reflects our own desire.

To live life in the here and now,
noble and upright,
let go that extra atom,
see the other side.
Expensive metals end in rust,
elements decline,
it's not the outer
but our soul
that will forever shine.
It's not what we can gain in life
but what we leave behind,
while winding back to Hydrogen,
the universal mind.[11]

References

1   Bohr N. On the Constitution of Atoms and Molecules. Parts I–III. *Philosophical Magazine* 1913; 26: 1–24, 476–502, 857–875.

2   Sherr J. *The Homeopathic Proving of Hydrogen.* Malvern: Dynamis Books; 1992.

3   Sherr J. Radioactivity – 50 years since Hiroshima and Nagasaki. *Homeopathic Links* 1995; 8(3): 10–11.

4   Wikepedia. Available online at: http://tinyurl.com/3xhj8t

5   Sherr J. *Dynamic Provings Volume I.* Surrey: Dynamis School; 1997.

6   Hahnemann CFS. *Organon of Rational Medicine*, 6th edition. (Dudgeon RE trans.) Philadelphia PA: Boericke and Tafel; 1896. §108.

7   Sharp HJ. The Octave and the Properties of the Elements, Endless Search – World Creation and Maintenance. Available online at: http://tinyurl.com/6ogzjbk

8   The Chakras, Mysticbeats.com website. Available online at: http://tinyurl.com/74ma48r

9   Wikipedia. Available online at: http://tinyurl.com/6k29y

10 Young AM. *The Reflective Universe*, Revised edition. Cambria CA: Anodos Foundation; 1999.

11 Sherr J. *Dynamic Materia Medica-Syphilis.* 2nd edition. Glasgow: Saltire Books; 2013.

part two

A DYNAMIC MATERIA MEDICA
HELIUM

1

INTRODUCTION

All religions, arts and sciences are branches of the same tree. All these aspirations are directed toward ennobling man's life, lifting it from the sphere of mere physical existence and leading the individual towards freedom.

Albert Einstein[1]

Homeopathic Helium

The initial proving of Helium was conducted in 1995 by the Dynamis School Norway and was later reproved by Silvie Gowan and friends in England. Further mini provings have followed. During that year I had the privilege of teaching five Dynamis courses concurrently in California, England, Holland, Israel and Norway. As a proving is an inherent part of every Dynamis course, I had to choose five different substances to prove. After a long search I managed to obtain a potency of Plutonium Nitricum. Naturally I felt very apprehensive about this proving. At the time no large-scale provings of a radioactive material had ever been conducted and certainly nothing with such an intimidating reputation as plutonium. I felt that it was only fair to ask the students if they were willing to prove a radioactive substance, without disclosing which one it was to be. I was sure none of the classes would agree.

To my surprise, when I approached the brave students of Dynamis Norway with this question, they agreed to do the radioactive proving. The following week I travelled to California and asked the same question. The California students also agreed. Later on, still apprehensive about this substance, I decided to do the Plutonium Nitricum proving in England, where I could supervise it more closely. I planned to do four other 'positive' provings to balance out the seemingly 'negative' Plutonium. I chose Olive (*Olea Europaea*) for Israel, Yew Tree (*Taxus Baccata*) for Holland, Bald Eagle (*Haliaeetus Leucocephalus*) for California and Helium for Norway. I had been planning to prove Helium for some time as I had already proved Neon and ultimately wanted to prove all the noble gases.

All of these provings were double-blind: Neither the provers nor the supervisors knew what the substance was, moreover provers were instructed not to talk to each other about the proving until it was over.

The interesting result of this unintentional experiment was that both the Norwegian group and the Californian group were under the definite impression they were proving a radioactive material. Yet surprisingly their provings in no way displayed any radioactive themes. On the contrary, a clear impression of Eagle emerged in the Haliaeethus proving, as did a clear image of Helium in the Helium proving. Neither proving contained any trace of radioactive imagery. One can thus deduce that knowing the proving substance does not necessarily bias a group of quality provers.

One curious symptom observed in the Helium proving was the distinct delusion of being an eagle. While there is a strong analogy between Eagle and Helium that could explain this symptom, I wondered, not for the first time, whether two provings conducted simultaneously could influence each other, even at a distance. I had seen the same phenomenon when the Salmon provers were convinced they had proved Wolf. Here again there is an analogy between wolves and salmon. However, the proving of Lac Lupinum was conducted in the United States at the same time as the salmon (*Oncorynchus tsawytscha*) proving was happening in England. This possible crossover may be explained in different ways: delusion, synchronicity, non-local effects and entanglement, the epidemic and sporadic nature of provings or the simple interconnectedness of the universe.

That being said, Helium has produced its own magic. It is certainly one of the most remarkable provings I have ever experienced. By the very nature of its location in the periodic table this proving touches on esoteric matters: God, the universe, our soul. It takes the mind to places where previously only imagination could carry us, to the mystery of mysteries, our origins.

The potencies of perception

In this book I equate the levels of perception in Helium with levels of potency. We can roughly compare the mother tincture level to the study of the material and chemical properties of the substance, while the higher potencies of perception penetrate the innermost nature of the remedy's simple substance. **This division into levels of potency is an analogy and has nothing whatsoever to do with the potencies taken by the provers or use in cases, it is merely an analogy to the depth of our understanding.**

Here is a brief summary of levels of potency equated with levels of perception, ranging from the gross to the subtle:

- The element itself represents purely chemical properties.
- The mother tincture represents homeopathic preparation and naturopathic use, the realm of atoms and molecules.
- The 12C level represents physical affinities, the realm of organs.
- The 30C represents general themes, the realm of the organism.
- The 200C represents essence, emotional pictures and signatures.
- The 1M and 10M potencies are an unravelling of the symptom configuration, a search for unified meaning in the totality.
- The 50M represents subtle sensations and functions, including the geometrical structure of the remedy.
- The CM explores the world of analogy and metaphor.
- The MM and beyond are an investigation into the esoteric roots of the remedy; the akashic records, cosmic library or the simple substance of Swedenborg and Kent.[i]

In my 'grammatical' method of analysis, the 12C and 30C represent nouns, the 200C and 1M are adjectives and adverbs while the 50M represents verbs, movement in time and space.[3] The potencies beyond transcend grammar as they touch the language of poetry.

Matching the remedy to the patient on the higher potencies of similarity will lead to deeper results, however for optimum similarity, all levels should fit.

I do not intend the correspondence of each potency level to a concept to be precise, rather a general idea. Creating yet another table or system to which homeopaths should rigidly adhere can only lead to an overcomplicated mode of thinking.

Please note that while I have ordered the following sections according to the potencies of perception, they are in no way related to the potency of prescriptions in cases or to the effects of proving potencies. This is merely an analogy. The sections on Helium 12c and Helium 30c in Chapter 3 do not relate to potency selection in prescribing, but to levels of perception. The potency should be selected according to the totality of the case regardless of the section in which it has been placed in this book.

---

[i] "The simple substance is the substance of substances, and all things are from it. It is really first, in which rests all power."[2]

Most Helium cases can be solved from knowledge gained from the 12C to the 50M levels of perception and I have included some examples of cases in Chapter 8. The higher levels of potency (CM and above) relate to simple substance and thus to broader concepts than the individual remedy. Not everyone will feel comfortable with the information in these high potency chapters. That is fine; there is no need to go there. I enjoy thinking of these things and maybe some readers will too. I intend to discuss the MMM and perhaps higher levels in the ultimate book on this series.

Only a few selected quotes from the provings have found their way into each section. Please be aware that it is important to read the proving as a whole to gain a thorough understanding of the remedy, as many symptoms only appear in the unabridged proving document, which is available online at www.thenoblegases.net

---

Recording of provings in the text

When capitalised, Helium and Hydrogen refer to homeopathic remedies, while helium and hydrogen in lower case refer to the basic elements.

All original symptoms from the Helium proving are given in blue type as follows: Helium symptom. Some proving symptoms have been abbreviated or grammar has been corrected without changing the essential content. Please bear in mind that the proving was translated from the Norwegian, hence the grammar may still sound awkward at times. The complete and original text can be found in the proving text itself.

Keywords and phrases that I consider important are occasionally marked **in bold** within the proving.

Reference

1   Einstein A. Moral Decay (1937), Essay in: *Out of My Later Years*. New York NY: Carol Publishing Group; 1995. pp 9–10.

2   Kent JT. *Aphorisms and precepts from extemporaneous lectures* (compiled by Carpenter HB). Chicago IL: Hahnemann, PP; 1897.

3   Sherr J. *The Dynamic Materia Medica – Syphilis*. 2nd edition. Glasgow: Saltire Books; 2013.

2

HELIUM THE ELEMENT

Discovery and naming

Helium was first discovered by French astronomer Pierre Janssen who visited India in 1868 to observe a full eclipse of the Sun. Janssen examined light from the sun with a spectroscope and was surprised to see some lines that could not be traced to any known element. He concluded that there must be an element on the sun that had never been seen on earth. Norman Lockyer observed the same eclipse and was the first to propose that the line was caused by a new element, which he named helium from the Greek word *helios* for sun.

For the next thirty years, chemists looked for helium on earth. In 1895, the English physicist Sir William Ramsay found helium in uranium. In 1907, Ernest Rutherford showed that an alpha particle of radiation is in fact a helium atom without its electrons, hence its presence in uranium.

Credit for the terrestrial discovery of helium is also attributed to Swedish chemists Per Teodor Cleve (1840–1905) and Nils Abraham Langlet, who discovered helium at about the same time in a mineral called cleveite. In 1903, large reserves of helium were found in natural gas fields in parts of the United States, which is by far the largest supplier of the gas.

Chemical properties of helium

Symbol: He
Atomic number: 2
Atomic mass: 4.002602

Helium is a colourless, odourless, tasteless gas. It is a member of the noble gas family: group 18 (VIIIA) of the periodic table. Next to hydrogen, it is the second most abundant element in the universe, and accounts for 24% of the elemental mass of our galaxy. The sun consists of 84% of hydrogen

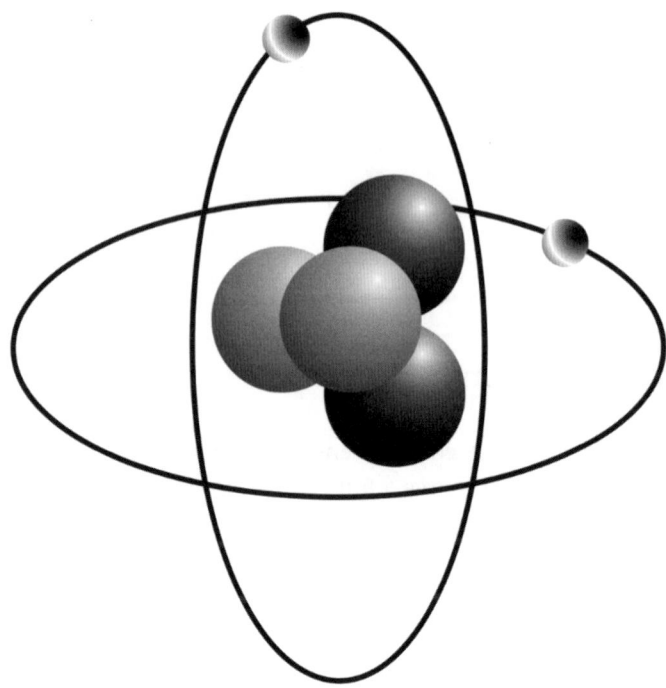

Figure 2.1 *Configuration of the Helium Atom*

atoms, 15% of helium atoms and only 1% of heavier atoms. Helium is formed in the sun's core by the fusion of hydrogen atoms.

All stars are formed by a process in which hydrogen fuses into helium. In this process six hydrogen atoms fuse into one helium atom. In the first step of the process, two hydrogen atoms fuse to form deuterium (an isotope of hydrogen with one extra neutron in its nucleus). In the next step, another hydrogen atom fuses with deuterium, creating a rare isotope of helium that has two protons and one neutron. In the third step, two rare helium atoms fuse to create a single normal helium atom and two 'left-over' hydrogen atoms. The net result is that four hydrogen atoms make up one helium atom (see Figure 2.1). The energy that fuels a star is a result of the difference in mass between the original four hydrogen atoms and the resulting helium atom. Following Einstein's mass-energy equivalence $E = mc^2$, the missing mass is converted into energy.

Helium has a number of unusual properties. For example, it has the lowest boiling point of any element: –268.9°C (–452.0°F). The freezing point of helium is –272.2°C (–458.0°F). Helium exists only as a gas except in extreme conditions and is the only gas that cannot be made into a solid simply by lowering the temperature. It stays in the liquid phase down to absolute zero and can only be transformed to solid phase under increased pressure (25atm).

At a temperature of about –271°C (–456°F), helium undergoes an extra-ordinary change into a superfluid. Superfluidity is a state in which matter behaves like a fluid without viscosity and with infinite thermal conductiv-ity. The substance, which appears to be a normal liquid, will flow without friction past any surface, which allows it to continue to circulate over obstructions and through pores in containers which hold it, subject only to its own inertia.[1] Since even gases have a degree of viscosity, superfluids have less resistance to shear than a gas. The forms of helium are so different that they are given different names: Above –271°C liquid helium is called helium I and below that temperature it is called helium II. Its physical prop-erties undergo a dramatic change. Helium II has such remarkable properties that it can justifiably be called a separate state of matter: the superfluid phase, in addition to the three classic phases (solid, fluid and gas).

Viscosity is greatly reduced in a superfluid. In comparison to usual liquids that become more viscous the lower the temperature, helium II becomes more fluid at lower temperatures. At 1K, helium II is about 100 times more fluid than at 2.19K. Superfluidity can be illustrated by the following experiment: helium II flows without friction at a speed of 22cm/s through a narrow capillary tube with a diameter of less than 0.01mm. If as much helium gas was to pass through the same capillary tube, it would take weeks compared to the seconds it takes helium II.

Helium is inflammable. With the exception of hydrogen, helium has the highest thermal conductive properties of all the gases. Its speed of diffusion through solid substances is only exceeded by hydrogen.

Uses of helium

Helium has a surprising number of applications for an inactive gas. It is used in low-temperature research, for filling balloons and dirigibles (blimps), to pressurise rocket fuels, in welding operations, lead detection systems, neon signs and to protect objects from reacting with oxygen.

The single most important use for helium is in low-temperature cooling systems. This is because liquid helium at –270°C is cold enough to cool anything else. One such use is in superconducting devices. These devices perform functions in the superconducting state that would be difficult or impossible to perform at room temperature. The superconducting state involves a loss of electrical resistance and occurs in many metals and alloys at temperatures near absolute zero.

Helium is used in the production of heliox air, a mixture of helium and oxygen in which the nitrogen in the air has been replaced by helium. Heliox is used by divers to speed up recovery from spinal decompression syndrome, also called the bends. On ascending from a dive, inert gas comes out of solution in a process called 'outgassing' or 'offgassing'. Under normal conditions, most offgassing occurs by gas exchange in the lungs. If an inert gas comes out of solution too quickly to allow outgassing in the lungs, then bubbles can form in the blood or within the solid tissues of the body, causing the symptoms. Like nitrogen, helium as an inert gas can cause the bends, but it is preferred because it does not cause narcosis.[2]

Compared to conventional air, heliox also offers certain advantages for the respiratory system and can give asthmatics considerable relief.

Helium: preparation of homeopathic potencies

The remedy was prepared by the Helios Pharmacy in England.

Pure helium gas (Sigma Aldrich UK Batch no 413001/1, 1994) was bubbled through pure water for 20 minutes. The solubility of helium is $0.94cm^3$ per 100ml of water. This resulting solution was considered to be a 1C. potency. It was then succussed and a 2C dilution was made in water. The water was to PhEur standard, ultra-purified by reverse osmosis.

Potencies up to 5C were similarly prepared in water and 90% organic grain ethanol (PhEur) was used for 6C and above.

References

1   Wikipedia. See: http://en.wikipedia.org/wiki/Superfluid
2   Wikipedia. See: http://en.wikipedia.org/wiki/Decompression_sickness

3

Helium 12C: Physical affinities

Helium affects every part of the body and it will require many clinical cases to assess its main affinities. From the proving I have observed strong affinities with the head and hair, skin and itching, throat, eyes, female and hormonal complaints including pregnancy, labour and ovaries, digestion and metabolism, vertigo, extremities, muscles, respiration, back and neck. For a list of physical symptoms, please refer to the full proving text at the end of this book.

Improvements noted from clinical cases include Delayed labour, premenstrual tension, neck and back pain, wandering pains, joints pains and digestive problems. For further reference see the cases in Chapter 8.

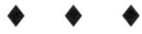

Helium 30C: Generalities

Some of the main general themes in Helium are sensations of floating and lightness or conversely heaviness accompanied by weight gain. Extreme energy versus extreme weakness, fatigue and indolence. Great restlessness, clumsiness, incoordination, chills, colds and bouts of flu, sensations of heat, constriction and pressure, stitching and twitching. Other themes include periodicity (weekly, yearly), as well as noon, evening and midnight modalities.

Helium 200C: Emotional Essence

We will begin our journey into the emotional realm of Helium with the more predictable aspects of the remedy. As one might expect from a noble gas that forms no chemical bonds, Helium provers experienced a sense of aloneness or isolation. Many provers felt a strong desire to be alone and undisturbed, and yearned for peace and quiet. They found a variety of ways to avoid company and to cut themselves off from the world, often hiding behind a book or shutting all the doors and windows. Many provers experienced an intense dislike of talking, touching or engaging in any social interaction, with a definite aversion to talking on the telephone. The feeling was one of "leave me alone, I don't need or want anyone". This isolation was often accompanied by apathy. The Helium patient may seem introverted, cold and distant to others. A useful clinical symptom appeared in one prover, who had a strong desire to go to an island or convent, which also reflects the religious aspect of Helium. They may spend a lot of time praying or meditating, and may have an affinity to religious music and healing.

The sense of separation might manifest as a calm tranquillity, as if not affected or touched by anything. A feeling of living in one's own world, calm, relaxed and not bothered by external circumstances. Even stressful situations such as car accidents left provers totally unmoved. This excessive calmness can tip over into total indifference, patients not wishing to be involved in any of their usual activities or having no feelings for loved ones. At its worst this evolves into stagnation, apathy and extreme lack of initiative. They are stuck in the world of plans and potential, yet cannot manifest any of it into action. A polarity of this apathy is a desire to read exciting stories and see action movies. Another polarity is sensitivity to others opinions, a sensation that people can see though them, and concern of what they will think.

Alongside the strong inclination to be alone and cut off from society, Helium patients may experience an overwhelming sense of loneliness, rejection and deep melancholy, a feeling that nobody cares. This may be accompanied by a desolate and depressed feeling, weepiness or a sense of vulnerability. Like many remedy provings, Helium produces irritability. What particularly characterises this irritability is a tremendous aversion to being disturbed. Any intrusion that penetrates their tightly closed shell aggravates, in particular noise. The following prover symptom serves as illustration:

Everything is irritating me, the way my friends talk, walk, eat, small sounds. Rage inside, wanting to hit everybody around me, to choke them. Everything inside me is grumpy, from my toes to the top. The grumpiness is **floating** inside me, as if boiling in my lungs; I want to scream at those around me. I want to be alone, not disturbed. It is a sour, deep, terrible feeling. (I am never normally irritated by anything.)

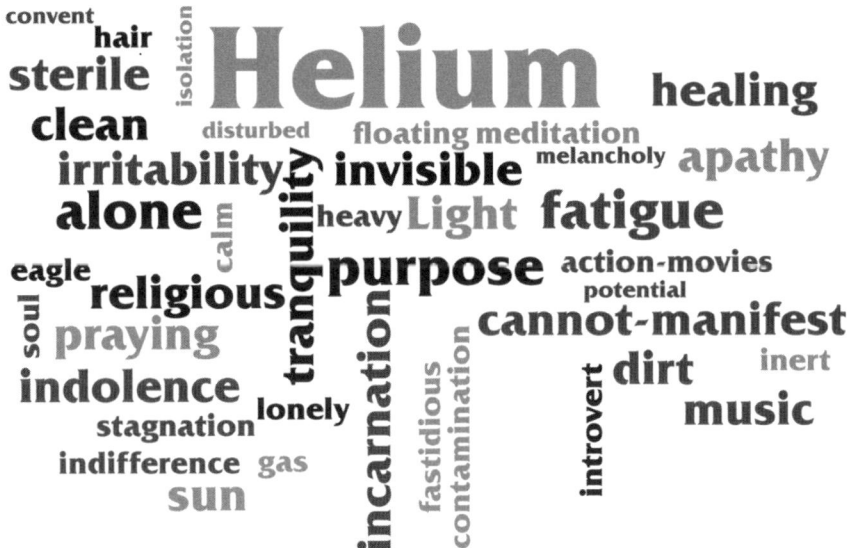

Figure 3.1 *An amalgamation of typical Helium themes*[1]

This irritability can develop into explosive anger over trifles. One prover had a desire to throw things, hit or even bite her child. Moods alternate between feeling positively cheerful and a violent, fighting rage.

An important theme is a great fastidiousness, especially regarding bodily cleanliness and in particular that of the hair. Helium patients may have an aversion to any dirt and possible contamination of their sterile world. Also prominent in the proving was a distorted sense of time, which seemed both fast and slow. For a pictorial representation of emotional themes see Figure 3.1.

◆ ◆ ◆

Helium 1M: Higher themes

An *up-down theme* is a common feature of most gases and Helium also shares this.

Heights

Helium can produce or cure a fear of heights. Some provers experienced a desire to go to the mountains and many had dreams of mountain to mountains, falling from mountain tops and aeroplanes. An unusual (and clinically confirmed) symptom was a desire to bounce up and down on a trampoline.

Dreamt one of my sons was walking on the edge of the veranda, there was no fence and it was a long way down. I was not afraid for him.

Floating sensation

Provers experienced sensations of floating and lightness, described by one prover as "a hydrogen feeling", as if his feet were not touching the ground. Another described a feeling of being a champagne bottle where the cork was just about to pop, with a strong current pushing up the spine.

Helium and hydrogen make up the first period of the periodic table. Hydrogen is lighter than air, floating out of the atmosphere and up into space. This manifested in the proving as a feeling of the soul leaving the body on its way to meet God. Though heavier than hydrogen, helium is still lighter than air.

A feeling as if my head were lighter, as if I were floating out into the universe.

Feeling as if I see myself from the outside, and from above.

The floating sensation of Helium differs from that of Hydrogen. While Hydrogen has a sensation of the soul leaving the body, in Helium the head feels light and the body feels heavy, fat and flabby. This is symbolic of the beginning of the soul entering or leaving the body. Due to the heaviness of helium relative to hydrogen, in Helium it is the head that separates rather than the soul.

I felt that my head was separated from my body: a very prominent feeling. Feeling of hard work to get my **head and body to fit together** again.

Dreamt I was going to the toilet which changed into an open lift. It went **straight up** and continued **upwards**, out of the building for hundreds of metres creating a tower as it went, then changed into a rocket. I only had a platform to stand on and I was very scared, **afraid of falling.** I could only look straight ahead. It felt like going **straight up into the sky**, to eternity. A force was pulling me by my **forehead and the top of my head**, so I felt **elongated**. At the same time a **fear of the altitude** in my stomach pulled me **heavier and heavier down toward the earth.** I felt a **split between my head and body,** located in the throat which was constricted, giving me a suffocated feeling with nausea as if I were **going to die.**

The eagle

A characteristic and strange expression of this upward theme is the distinct sensation of being an eagle.

I feel sharp-sighted, as if I can see through things. Like a hunting animal, an eagle. I can see details at a long distance, and as if from above, high up. I saw a sheep and thought about attacking it.

This eagle sensation was accompanied by a feeling of having acute vision and of looking at the world from above, both physically and emotionally. There were feelings of aloofness and superiority, a great clarity of vision, as well as the ability to penetrate or 'see through' others.

I can see the details of the surroundings very clearly, both mentally and physically. I feel that I can 'see' the children.

My eyes feel clearer and I can look at other people more directly. I feel my eyes penetrating when looking at others, while my mind is safe and secure. Other people can't touch me. I have a very strong core.

Many mineral remedies have animal analogies hidden within them. This is why the doctrine of signatures approach (i.e. elephant sensation equals elephant remedy) represents an unsophisticated level of homeopathy. Through provings we learn to see the correspondences that transcend kingdom classification. There are many similarities between gas remedies (such as Ozone) and birds, and Helium and the eagle are a particularly good example. Both are noble, both avoid mixing with the world, both feel superior and fly high up in the sky. The eagle is the king of birds, while Helium wears the crown of the periodic table. Both are associated with *helios*, the sun, and both remedies share the delusion that there are two suns in the sky. The circumscribed white head of the bald-headed eagle reflects the head-body split of Helium. Many emotional themes of Helium are reminiscent of those of *Haliaeetus Leucocephalus*: looking from above, a desire to be alone in the mountains, a floating sensation, indifference, tranquillity, penetrating vision, alone and isolated, alternating moods and explosive anger. Even the names Helium and *Haliaeetus* reflect the similarity.

I had an image of Thor Heyerdahl. He was an **eagle**, looking like an eagle, **seeing things from above**, revealing the pattern of how people travelled in ancient times. I thought he looked **cold** and I felt sorry for him. What would it be like to be so cold? I thought of things I have read about his childhood: that he felt **separated from his environment**, something in his upbringing, no play. His mother was into Darwinism and practical, **down to earth** things, while his father **believed in God** and told him stories from the Bible.

This image illustrates more about Helium than just the eagle. From the lofty peaks of the periodic table, Helium perceives the big picture yet remains detached from it all in noble isolation. The contrasting characters of Thor Heyerdahl's parents reflect two of the contrasting polarities in Helium: being down to earth as opposed to deeply religious.[i]

God, healing and music

Spirituality and a yearning for God are important aspects of Helium. This is more of a spiritual longing then religious ritualistic behaviour. While Hydrogen has only just separated from God, Helium has taken the first step away from the creator towards earthly existence and the gap has widened. Meditating for long periods of time, chanting or praying in church were some of the experiences shared by the provers. From the original proving language you can sense the difference between Hydrogen's universal soul and Helium's individual soul, longing and praying for reconnection with the divine.

Longing to be one with God. I got palpitations like when you're in love when I thought about it. It is a sad longing, a wistfulness. I sat down to meditate, but felt a stronger need to kneel down and pray, to send my wishes out. Desire to be in touch with God, near God.

Other aspects of Helium's spirituality include a strong love of music, especially new-age, spiritual music, church music or Bach. Helium also has

---

[i] Thor Heyerdahl is famous for the Kon-Tiki expedition. He organised and led a 1947 expedition from Peru to Polynesia on the balsa raft Kon-Tiki to demonstrate the possibility of aboriginal South American voyages to the Oceanic islands.

a remarkable ability to see people's auras, as well as an intense capacity for healing and transmitting energy. Healing, whole, healthy, helios, Helium.

Feeling a strong healing power in my hands, starting to treat patients with healing.

Helium patients may have a desire to shave their head, which relates to the Helium effect on the crown chakra. It is as if they want their crown to be totally open to the sky.

Desire to shave all the hair off my head.

My hair caused constant irritation. I felt like cutting it off short-short. I had to tie it up into a ponytail to keep it away from my face.

The Helium desire to shave the head, pray, chant or go to a monastery indicates that Helium may be a good remedy for monks, Hare Krishna devotees and a whole variety of new-age disciples. This hypothesis has been clinically verified.

Obsessive compulsive disorder

As we might expect from a noble gas proving, Helium is prone to extreme perfectionism. Shaving the head is one example of this. Any hair that is dirty or out of place becomes a source of irritation. This perfectionism can easily become an obsessive compulsive disorder, especially regarding cleanliness, washing and germs. In opposition to this fanatical cleanliness are dreams of dirt. To Helium the physical world is filthy and polluted and they would rather remain in their own uncontaminated isolation.

I took a shower and took a long time to clean every single hair on my head and every part of my body.

Strong desire to have the house tidy and clean, feeling it looks dirty.

Feel a need to protect myself mentally from the germs in the breath of a sick child. I felt he had dirty, offensive breath, even though it wasn't really. I didn't want to have his 'uncleanliness' in myself.

I dreamt that my flat was very dirty (earth/mud), especially the bathroom. The bathroom floor was covered with beetles that were difficult to get rid of. They bit my **big toe**. When I touched them they were soft and like dog shit. My main feeling was: My flat is so dirty and I couldn't manage to keep it clean.

As we already hypothesised, the noble gift of perfect existence is also Helium's Achilles heel. Perfectionism wraps Helium in an isolating layer, preventing contact with the grimy joys of life in this world.

Dreamt that there was something wrong with my skin. An outer layer was sick and I needed an operation to get rid of it. But I found that I could peel off a thick layer myself, easily and without pain. Inside there was fresh new skin, all clean and perfect.

In the shower I had a revelation that things are not perfect, you can't be too idealistic, you have to accept or else you get cold and cynical. (curative)

During the proving I was cold and observing. I felt no joy, My heart was not with things

Helium 10M: Spiritual themes

In Helium 10M the two prominent themes of Helium, that of being high up and that of purity versus filth combine into one idea. Living outside the body, or rather body in and head out, Helium cannot bear to enter a dirty and contaminated reality. The price she must pay for this purity is to remain out of touch with the world, a soul unwilling to undertake incarnation.

A curious phenomenon in the Helium proving is that many of the dreams of dirt versus cleanliness take place on mountain tops, reflecting the pristine and lofty position of the unincarnated Helium soul.

In our cottage in the **mountain**s I see a mouse crossing the floor. The place is not clean; it is **untidy** and not very well maintained. It doesn't feel like a safe place to sleep in. Outside it is very **green and nice** with a lovely river.

Swimming in **muddy water** with an old boyfriend and my daughter in the **mountains**. It is unpleasant and uncomfortable. Then new **clear water** comes and it turns into a pool.

Dreamt of being **high up in the mountains** with a lot of snow. Three cows are coming up the side of the hill. A pile of **newly washed clothes** is lying in the snow. The clothes are white and green. My son was with me and I asked him to hurry, since I was afraid that the smell of the cows would **contaminate** the clothes.

Soon after the proving I was reading a book called *Journey of Souls* by Dr Michael Newton.[2] Rather than taking his patients back to a past life, Dr Newton, a hypnotherapist, developed techniques to journey with them to the place between lives, documenting their impressions of the afterlife. While in a state of deep hypnosis, twenty-nine people recalled their experiences as spirits between incarnations on earth. Dr Newton believes that the hypnotic responses of his subjects concerning the afterlife provide credible information because of the consistency of their reports. Patients often used the same words and graphic descriptions. These descriptions include accounts on how it feels to die, who meets us after death, where we go and what we do as souls, different levels of souls, why we choose to come back in certain bodies and how we learn to recognise our soul mates on earth. More importantly, the subjects describe how souls learn from the mistakes of past lifetimes and consequently choose the setting and purpose of their next life.

Whether you believe Dr Newton's findings to be fact, fiction, imagination or fabrication makes little difference. What is important for our purpose is that its collective imagery resonates strongly with the proving of Helium, helping us to understand the remedy's inner nature. I have solved many cases with the help of this understanding, thus giving some degree of validity to this association.

For the purpose of illustrating the remedy, I will compare the Helium proving with accounts of the soul's journey between incarnations as documented by Dr Newton.

The soul's journey

Books such as *Life after Life* by Dr Raymond Moody describe people's accounts of near-death experiences.[3] They tell of the soul leaving the body, floating upwards, travelling through a narrow tunnel and arriving at a place described as the "light of a million suns" or a meeting with God. Several remedies (such as Thuja, Anacardium and Sabadilla) have a sense of leaving the body, but these relate to the earlier stages of this journey. Descriptions of the end stage of this journey are more analogous to cannabis-indica and especially Hydrogen:

I felt odd, as if I was hardly in my body. Feel like my body is working on automatic but I'm not really there. Driving along I kept forgetting where I was. Now I feel I'm really more 'absent' than normal and feel quite afraid of losing my mind or having an accident. I feel my connection with the physical world is very loose, as though my soul were separated from my body. I have thoughts that this is a bit like dying – not unpleasant.

From the proving of Hydrogen

I felt in the presence of a totally pure energy, like meeting God and feeling totally unworthy or like meeting a lover and feeling unworthy – realising all the mistakes of a lifetime.

From the proving of Hydrogen

The light I was seeing was brighter than I had ever seen before.

From the proving of Helium

It felt as if my body had disappeared, I tried to feel it, but couldn't. As if it didn't belong to me, as if it wasn't there.

From the proving of Helium

Now we venture one step further into the soul's journey. The next step of the death process as related by Dr Newton is more analogous to the Helium proving. Hypnotised patients describe how souls float upwards, shining in different aura colours according to their state of spiritual evolution. Here are the Helium provers' accounts:

I see light around people, the light is moving, sometimes flashing strongly, also colours.

I see things clearer, also a light aura around some people. Some are stronger than others and sometimes they flash all over the place.

I felt it was all about returning to the force of light. I kept seeing halos and auras, like everything was joined together and was all light, everything merged and no space in between.

Dreamt I wanted to give light to everybody.

According to Dr Newton, souls proceed to join their groups, which are clusters of energy that appear like transparent bubbles or translucent bulbs. They contain entities who often shared past lives.

Dreamt about old friends, meeting them and then losing them and ending up on my own. It was quite a nice time. I was in the mountains.

I went into a hotel and took the lift quite high up and went into a room where two ladies were present. All of us had the impression that we had experienced this situation long ago. We tried to find out when it could have been.

Dreamt I was back working as a tourist guide in Rome. Suddenly I saw an old friend standing outside, bathed in sunlight. I ran to her, and as we hugged and laughed I felt extreme joy and happiness, it was like being a child again.

Back to school

As a part of restoration after a lifetime on earth, souls enter a place of healing. This can be visualised as a school-type building, often in the form of a temple, where they are sent to examine their past lives together.

I had a vision of a golden temple with dark water surrounding it (see Figure 3.2).

Dreamt about the cathedral in Oslo. It disappeared like a cloud dissolving and behind it appeared an older church or holy place built from yellow stone with many windows and portals, standing on a grass green hill.

Thinking for several days about my dream of 'holy water' and becoming initiated. What does it mean to my life right now? I get the feeling it is from long ago, from another life.

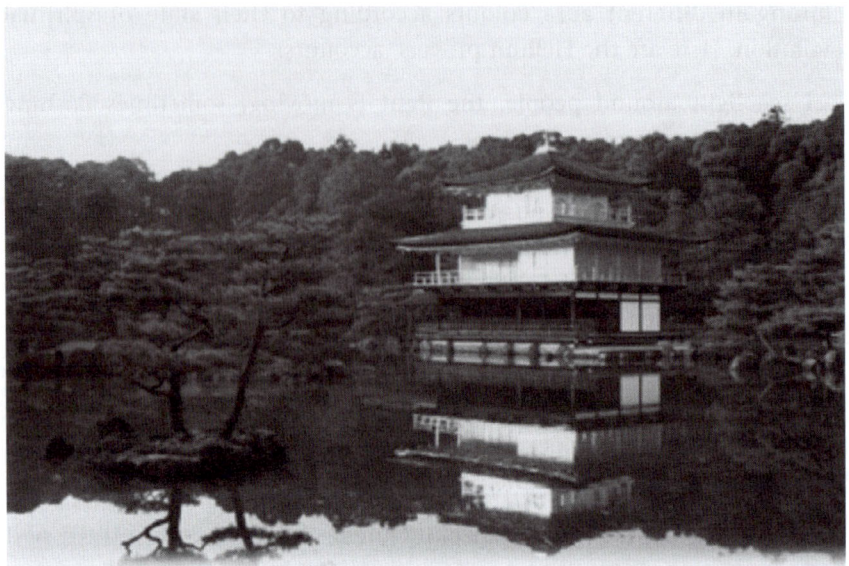

Figure 3.2 *Kinkaku-ji or Temple of the Golden Pavilion (also known as Rokuon-ji) is a Zen Buddhist temple in Kyoto, Japan*

Dr Newton goes on to explain how all souls have a personal guide who may be with them throughout many lives. Soul groups usually have leaders or spirit guides of a more advanced level. A life review is conducted, first with the spirit guides and later with a council of elders. Here the soul examines its last incarnation and mistakes that have been made during the past lifetime. There is no sense of judgment or criticism, it is merely a process of reviewing and learning.

As if I had dreamt I had done it all before. It felt we were never given more than we were ready for. Remembering and not wanting to repeat mistakes. Only fully loving if giving and receiving.

Dreamt about a beautiful black prostitute thinking about her life. I could see her thoughts. She feels like she has been cheating and treating many people badly, doing the same selfish things over and over again.

Suddenly I can see how I am similar to my father. I am aware of things in myself that I don't like in him. I see myself in a very direct way, as if from the outside, with no holds barred.

I was really aware of the Star Brethren walking beside me – I could literally see them as if they were physical! They were huge beings, 12 feet or so high, in wonderful white-gold robes. I could have stooped and touched their robes, and they were striding along beside me!

As souls learn and improve through their incarnations, they advance to higher and higher levels.

As soon as you accomplish one level, you are presented with another.

Dreams about finding the innate energy pattern of each person in order to help heal them or reactivate their energies. So having to delve beneath their symptoms and characteristics, and not be taken in by these, instead seeking the deep, inner energy pattern. The whole dream was like an adventure; like seeking the Holy Grail and having to go through many tests and adventures to ultimately get to the Grail.

According to Dr Newton, souls go to a place of life selection to examine alternative future lives to lead. The coming incarnation is chosen according to what they need to learn.

I feel like I am going before the Great Lords of Karma and tentatively and nervously saying that I am ready to go forward to my next set of karmic tests, into my next human life.

As an individual, you make your choice and then you become part of the whole and lose your individuality.

Dreamt I was staying at some sort of huge conference centre with our usual holiday group. The entrance doorway was different to how it would normally be and I could not work out how to get through it and out. **Then every time I did go through it, I came out a different** way and went through different corridors. It was a bit like a maze really.

A sense that my work situation is returning full circle in order for that cycle to end fully and another one begin. As if it cannot be as it used to be and something new is required.

Won't come in

What goes up must come down and eventually the soul must return to a body. However the Helium patient's soul is reluctant to come back into life and to engage with all its difficulties. It prefers the comfortable and pristine environment of heaven. There can be several reasons for this. Either it is repulsed by the dirt, grime and imperfection of the real world or it senses lurking dangers. We can compare this feeling to that of a child from a privileged background on her first day at a school in a rougher area of town.

Sensation of being very immature, not yet ready to be in this world.

It felt like my soul is reluctant to inhabit a body – a reluctance.

It felt like the world was not pure enough. Too open an impression to all possibilities so I have to withdraw. Too much impurity.

Dream of going to a house to adopt a beautiful baby girl. I noticed her falling in slow motion but it was a soft landing. As I picked her up, she said, "Hi". The mother said my lap was too hot to put her on.

Dreamt that I was walking through a dangerous part of a big city at night, carrying a handbag and a heavy suitcase. I was in several dangerous situations over a long period of time. I could only trust myself, everybody else was a potential enemy planning to assault me.

Another reason for the soul's reluctance to enter the world may be the fear of being criticised in the earthly realm. This stands in stark contrast to the heavenly state of examination without judgment.

It is like taking a new step forward and not being sure where that will take me and what people will think of it.

As if it is somehow about a Brave New Order and having to be brave to step forward, even though you are nervous about it because you haven't attempted it before and what will people think.

It is like actually realising your dreams and fantasies, but in front of others somehow and worrying that you will be criticised.

One of the impurities of this world with which Helium struggles is any form of dishonesty. For Helium people, everything must be in direct alignment with the vertical axis of truth. It is impossible to flex into fabrication or deal with the impurity of lies. Even a white lie appears contaminated. As most of humanity exists on a diet rich in lies, avoiding them altogether can prove very difficult. To put it another way, Helium patients have no idea how to play the game of life.

Distress at seeing people lying (not telling the truth).

Felt I was unsure, I only wanted to write truth not duality and I was not sure I wanted to join in with life.

I didn't want to be lied to anymore. I feel I have no true friends, no one is speaking the truth.

Felt I didn't understand the rules of life – the game of life. I wasn't sure whether I was here or just observing, not part of the game of life.

This reluctance to return to the body cannot keep the soul in a suspended state of pre-incarnation forever. According to Dr Newton, souls are not required to reincarnate, however considerable pressure is brought to bear on them by the spirit guides when the time is right. One part of the soul must join a new living foetus, while a **dormant part of the soul remains in heaven during every incarnation.**

Here is one remarkable dream from the proving of Helium:

While participating in the proving, I had a powerful dream that left a great impression on me. I dreamt that I was climbing up a steep mountain path with a group of friends and a leader. When we reached the top we were supposed to jump off. It was very high, about three miles up. It was like jumping from a plane. I was scared but eventually I jumped. It was a beautiful scene. I floated down easily and it was very enjoyable. We ascended again and this time gathered in a small house on the mountain top where there were naked dolls – empty shells with some bits of dolls strewn around. We had to jump and I was scared again, but this time there was water rising from below. We could wait for the water to ascend to the top of the mountain for an easy jump, or just take the risk and jump now.

In light of Dr Newton's findings, this dream may symbolise the ascendancy of a soul to a higher place of learning, followed by its descent to reincarnate on earth. The shock of incarnation is described as being more intense than death, so it is no wonder that jumping seemed so scary in the dream. Dr Newton goes on to describe how the soul can leave and re-enter the foetus's body several times during pregnancy. In the dream, descending the second time was much easier because of the rising water, analogous to the water filling the uterus. The dolls can be interpreted as bodies which the soul can choose.

All this may seem strange and if it does not fit your belief system, consider it as a metaphor. However, it is interesting to juxtapose the aforementioned dream with the following symptoms from two other provers:

Dreams of old dolls in attics.

Dreamt I was on a grass-covered, pointed hilltop with my sister. She was falling down, but I got hold of her and pulled her up again.

Dream that my girlfriend and I were both pregnant, very visibly so. One of the party games was to climb ladders (like gym wall exercise ladders).

Coming in

Eventually the Helium soul has no choice but to incarnate and undertake the journey back into the body. From a 'healthy' noble gas standpoint, the return of the soul to its body will be ideal, resulting in a perfect being.

A beautiful dream full of shining light and love in which I gave birth to a baby boy. Holding him in my arms I knew that the love I felt for him was endless and unconditional. Everybody came to see him; everybody loved him because he was pure goodness. He started to talk and we all knew that he was a miracle, like Jesus Christ. He had a pure shining glow around him. When I woke up I had such a feeling of happiness that I was almost floating.

I was in some Japanese-inspired surroundings. An egg-shaped pond with ice-cold water, and a thin layer of ice on top. I didn't know if it was muddy or full of plants, fishes, other creatures or anything dangerous. I undressed completely and jumped in after a short hesitation. The others around thought it was a great, impressive, respectful thing to do. My body broke the ice as I jumped into the pool. The water was ice-cold but clear. I went all the way to the bottom and then rose slowly upwards. The sun was shining through the water making all the bubbles glitter. I had to take a deep breath while still under water and found that I could breathe in the water. When I broke through the top it was like going through a membrane. I rose from the pond feeling like a new person, a cleaned person, actually more 'me' than ever. I was in contact with all of myself, and felt very whole. It felt like an initiation and I was met with deep respect afterwards.

For most souls, however, the process of leaving the source is a sad and painful one. While we all go through this process once a lifetime, the Helium patient remains stuck in this grief-stricken place.

Sadness at having to be born again, sad leaving where I had come from.

More and more awareness about us all being souls of light and that we come down into the narrow structure and restraints that incarnation and karmic conditions bring.

As if I am preparing for something that I haven't done before.

Groups

As Dr Newton's patients testify, just prior to incarnation family, partners, friends and enemies are chosen (reminding us of the children's game: 'I'll be the Daddy and you can be the Mummy'). They agree on identifying signs with which to recognise each other (i.e. you will come off the bus wearing a red hat or you will have a crooked little finger). Once the souls incarnate into life they must keep in contact with their group and play out the game.

This remedy is about re-grouping into a group with people you really want to be with and who are really on the same path as you.

I have an image of a school sports team and choosing the sides you want to be on, and changing sides at the last minute as you realise you would in fact rather be on the other team. A sense that this is the eleventh hour when you finally have to choose where your allegiance lies and whom it is with.

Question: Was I ready to honour the pact I had made in my previous lifetime?

Purpose

We now arrive at the crux of Helium's spiritual characteristics, one that has guided me to prescribe this remedy in many cases with excellent results. When the soul has finished its learning process, it decides how to spend its next lifetime and the purpose of its forthcoming incarnation. When in health, our life mission will be clear and will be achieved in the course of our lifetime.

As our fontanelles close and harden, we lose our direct (vertex, vertical) connection to heaven and our purpose is forgotten. Most people go through life oblivious of any sense of purpose and hence are merely surviving. Of the few that remember a sense of purpose and can recognise what it is, only a handful can claim they have achieved it fully. In health our life events are experienced in the right sequence, time and place. We die and are reborn in the time and place of our destiny, we live our purpose without dwelling on it and we achieve our life's mission.

One of the main characteristics of the Helium patient is a constant dwelling on life's purpose and destiny. It may be an awareness of having lost touch with their mission in life or a grief over not having achieved it. While the great majority of people will remain mostly unaware of this issue, it is a prominent and recurring obsession with Helium patients.

I have been thinking a lot about my destiny, where I belong, where my place is. I feel I haven't yet reached it.

Feeling hopeless about my future, that my work is of no use to anyone.

Dream: A friend's husband came home. I felt afraid that she did not need my help any more. My feeling was one of loneliness, and I wondered about the purpose of my life.

Dream: A glass of holy water was standing on the table on my right. I was going to drink this to be initiated to start my mission. Before drinking it I hugged my dear boyfriend who looked like Jesus. We both had tears in our eyes, knowing that now my mission was the main thing in my life.

It felt like everybody forgot the game because they were so absorbed that they forgot their purpose.

My way of praying changed from "God, please do this . . ." to "God, please help me to accept what happens".

My feelings of being alone with it all are uppermost or magnified. How being a homeopath basically means you are alone with a lot of responsibility. Feeling that I am not doing enough for some of my patients, that I do not deserve to have a good reputation.

Again this lonely feeling. It's about the purpose of my life. Things come to the surface. There seems to be something I'm finishing in my life. The remedy opens up and closes down. I now feel very good.

It made me realise that I feel I have achieved all my dreams and desires and do not have anything else to strive for at present. I have desired to be a spiritual, intuitive person from an early age. I have desired to be a healer and a homeopath, run my own practice and make a living from it. I have desired to have kids; I have desired a settled, loving relationship. All the things that I have desired and striven for, I have achieved. But now where do I go? I feel I have come to a full stop. I have no more dreams, hopes or fantasies left, and my life as it is now no longer feeds me. My work situation no longer feeds or inspires me.

I feel as if I don't want to waste any time. I only want to do important things, no unnecessary conversation. (curative)

Much less bad conscience about what I do and what people think about me. I don't have to do things. I feel much more free to make my own choices, so I am not so tied up by all the 'musts'. (curative)

I see more clearly what is my responsibility and what is other people's. (curative)

Maybe I am at the stage of letting go of desire, of my will. I am going through the process of following my heart and working more from the will of God; the experience, not just the knowledge of spiritual truth. Yet it is still all to do with work, direction, life purpose and what you achieve as an individual. (curative)

Hahnemann: a sense of purpose

The Helium preoccupation with life's mission reminds me of our great master, Christian Friedrich Samuel Hahnemann, the founder of homeopathy. Hahnemann is one of the few people who not only realised his purpose in life, but through hard work, genius, devotion and love, achieved his noble mission. The following two aphorisms from the *Organon* show the importance Hahnemann put on realising and fulfilling the soul's purpose.[4]

> The physician's **high and only mission** is to restore the sick to health, to cure, as it is termed (§1).

In the **healthy condition of man**, the spiritual vital force (autocracy), the dynamis that animates the material body (organism), rules with unbounded sway, and retains all the parts of the organism in admirable, harmonious, vital operation, as regards both sensations and functions, so that our indwelling, reason-gifted mind can freely employ this living, healthy instrument for the **higher purposes of our existence** (§9).

And the following from *Chronic Diseases*:[5]

If I did not know for what purpose I was put here on earth – to become better myself as far as possible and to make better everything around me, that is within my power to improve . . .

Finally on Hahnemann's grave, the short yet poignant epitaph:
Non inutilis vixi (I have not lived in vain).

Inertia/action

In the disease state the Helium patient is out of alignment with his mission, not fulfilling life's purpose and thus cut off from the source of energy and enthusiasm. Consequently he is left feeling empty, inert, directionless and confused:

I felt that I wasn't able to do things I was supposed to do; a feeling of failure. The heavy feeling prevented me from doing it, I neglected my duty.

I don't grab the opportunities the day brings. I want to withdraw from all duties, also from all spiritual work.

I felt very tired and did what I had to do without joy and enthusiasm.

I don't have much enthusiasm for anything. I'm bored, heavy and just want to sleep.

I'm considering whether my usual way of doing several things at the same time could be the cause of my fatigue and stress.

Stasis, stasis, stasis. Which is the worst thing for a Gemini like me! I wish I could break free. Everyone is moving and changing except for me.

At work I feel very bored and flat about it. Is this all my life is going to be?

I am just extremely bored and disinterested with work. I always love the 'chase' of finding a remedy, but I am also bored. Day after day of this sedentary occupation listening to other people's stories.

Helium patients can become quite wearisome, even to themselves. They exist in a constant state of potential without the ability to translate thoughts into action. They may have difficulty manifesting any plans. Some examples I have seen in practice were an architect who designed the perfect house but never built it, or a writer who was full of ideas for books but never wrote any. They may be stuck in a loop of thought that goes round and round in their head in an obsessive way, for instance counting the number plates on cars.

Never feeling like I'm quite ready. It feels like the 'how' is missing. I need to create rather than passively observe. Time for action really.

During the proving it feels as if I have more thoughts and less instincts.

I feel like everyone is a potential friend. Passive with potential but no action as yet.

Realisations that help you see more clearly about a situation, so that instead of being frustrated and impatient, you know that you have to wait or know what action you need to take.

In this inert state, disconnected from his soul's purpose and lacking enthusiasm, Helium lives in a meaningless and apathetic state. He exists in potential intention, unable to manifest his destiny. The only way to galvanise this inactive noble gas into action is by pumping it with electrical energy. Thus the Helium patient may crave action to revitalise his missing spark.

One night I drove through a red light several times (which I have never done before) and only felt **excited** and in control, the king of the road!

Feeling like doing something **exciting** like checking into a hotel under a false name.

I wanted to sing and dance and **do something crazy**. I drove the car like mad, singing at the top of my voice.

I wanted to **do something crazy**, to run and dance but not together with my boyfriend.

I wanted to watch an **action movie** so I rented one. I never wanted to do that before but it happened several times during the proving.

I went to see an **action movie** at the cinema. Not enough action for me, I wanted more. I wanted to see another one straight away.

Saw an **action movie** and thoroughly enjoyed it, I found it refreshing.

I spent the evening reading a book for young teenagers. **Exciting, action**, I couldn't stop reading. I had palpitations from the **excitement**.

I only want to speak about important matters. I don't make telephone calls to my friends. I'd rather help them through **actions** rather than words.

I am getting lots of things **done quickly.** Reflecting on this it seems to be that the weight of dragging around so much stuff that is not of the present moment slows things down.

I wondered initially how the electrical current that lights up the noble gases would surface in the proving. The desire for action in Helium could be analogous to the spark of energy that galvanises us into life.

Conclusion to Helium 10M Spiritual level

It is important to understand that while we have described the soul's journey of incarnation as an analogy to the Helium proving, in practice this will manifest as pathology, meaning that the Helium patient can become stuck in any one of the phases of soul evolution. A healthy living human being should not be seeing himself from above, living in 'stuck' perfection, or constantly musing on the purpose of his existence.

Just as helium is the only element that cannot become solid even at absolute zero, the Helium soul cannot incarnate into a physical body. Helium patients cling to their lofty position on the vertical line of static perfection, avoiding the reality of life. They refuse to lean forward and take the plunge into grimy existence. One cannot live life to the full by avoiding its contaminated reality. Rather we should engage with our grubby, lie infested world, and through faith, love and hard work transform it back into purity. If we remain at home because of a fear of school, we will never learn.

Some salmon never leave their birthplace in the cool, clear mountain springs, never swim downstream and out to the salty seas. The dangers are simply too great. However they will never experience the great journey, or realise their destiny by struggling upriver to spawn. In order to potentise ourselves to a higher level of being, it is not enough to enjoy the dilution of the noble gases. We must experience the painful succussion of life as we struggle upstream towards our noble quest.

References

1   www.wordle.com

2   Newton M. *Journey of Souls: Case Studies of Life Between Lives*. Woodbury MN: Llewellyn Publications; 1994.

3   Moody RA. Life After Life: *The Investigation of a Phenomenon – Survival of Bodily Death*. Seattle WA: Mockingbird Books; 1975. p. 175.

4   Hahnemann CFS. *Organon of Rational Medicine*, 6th edition. (Dudgeon RE trans.) Philadelphia PA: Boericke and Tafel; 1896.

5   Hahnemann, CFS. (Hempel, C. trans.) *The Chronic Diseases, their Specific Nature and Homoeopathic Treatment 1828*, New York NY: William Radde; 1845.

4

HELIUM 50M:
SENSATION, FUNCTION, STRUCTURE

Seeing from above

We will now examine the vertical axis of Helium and the other noble gases and how this idea emerges in the proving picture. The following is an interesting Helium symptom, which is similar to symptoms that occur in some of the other noble gases:

I had the sense that all my limbs felt foreshortened, my head and eyes were huge, I felt I had eyes all over my head, all-seeing. I felt withdrawn and my limbs felt short.

There is only one perspective from which we see the body as short-limbed and in 360 degrees, and that is from a vertical line directly above our vertex. The vertex is the 'death canal', the point between the fontanels through which the soul enters and departs from the body. Helium is viewing life from directly above this point. From this position everything below appears shorter and we can see in all directions, perceiving ourselves and others from a higher place in both a physical and spiritual sense. When light shines from directly above us there can be no shadow side.

Feels as if I see myself from the outside, and from above.

I feel very tall as though I am towering over everything.

I feel very tall so when I look down it is as if everything were a long way off.

I see myself in a very direct way, as if from the outside, with no holds barred. It feels as if I have more judgment, clarity, perspective and I am more sharp-sighted. I feel superior.

I saw myself from the outside. I was working at a lot of different places. I went swimming and was jumping from 10-metre heights.

I see things very clearly, how things really are.

My boyfriend was really 'seeing' me. I was 'naked' the whole weekend, showing sides of myself that I normally hide.

I felt 'naked' and very embarrassed that other people could see me in this situation.

In the morning waking up with a special clarity, as if seeing myself from the outside. I see situations in relation to people objectively, from the outside.

I can see the details of my surroundings very clearly, both mentally and physically. I feel I can 'see' the children.

The vertical axis of life on which Helium is situated runs from mid-heaven, through the vertex of the head, down the spine, out through the perineum and down to mid-earth. This is the line of the noble gases, the spine of the periodic table. It is the central axis around which a healthy, non-psoric person revolves, being in the perfect position rather than having a *dis*position.

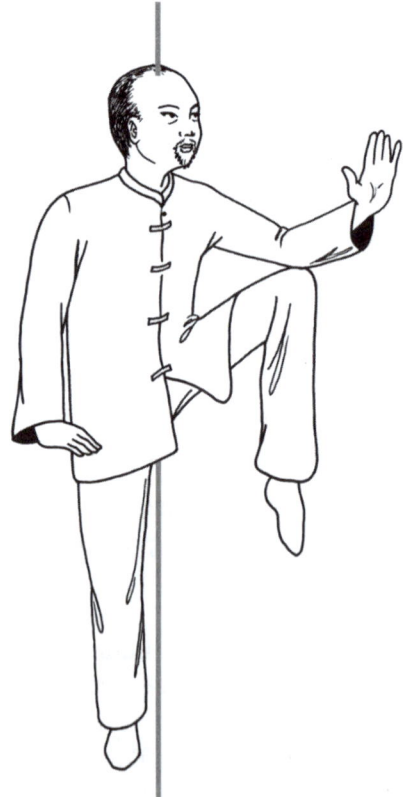

Figure 4.1 *This dynamic, vertical alignment is what the T'ai Chi master seeks*
(Graphic by Brenda Brown www.odesk.com)

This dynamic, vertical alignment is what the T'ai Chi master seeks (see Figure 4.1). When we are aligned we are 'in the zone', flowing in synchronicity with the universe. This noble axis is the line of truth, love and wisdom, where all things happen at the right time and in the right place. It is the line of here and now and therefore it is the line of health. Heaven and earth flow through us, so that we no longer need to expend our own energy. Therefore we do not decay.

> If even heaven and earth must rest,
> How much more so human beings?
> Therefore align yourself to the Way.
> Aligned with the Way you are one with the Way.
> Aligned with virtue you are one with virtue.
> Aligned with the heavens you are one with the heavens.
> The Way accepts this alignment gladly.
> Virtue accepts this alignment gladly.
> The heavens accept this alignment gladly.
>
> *Tao Te Ching* by Lao-Tsu[1]

I felt I could do and change anything in the whole world by **aligning myself with that love** and bringing it into any and every situation in my life. I felt very purposeful.

There are several Helium symptoms that relate to curling up, opposite to the vertical alignment. This theme of deviating from the straight line or curling up also emerges in the other noble gases.

I woke shocked awake, because I was lying straight in the bed. **Curling up** on my back ameliorated.

I was finding it hard to breathe when I was stretched out, so **curling around ameliorated.**

I **curl up** on my back.

Delusion that I was trussed up. My wrists tied to my ankles, my legs between my thighs, lying on my side.

Thoughts felt like knots of worms.

Shadows

When Helios the sun shines from its highest zenith at noon it creates no shadows. While Helium is in an 'out of body' state, she views herself from directly above and in all directions.

Delusion that I had a large head covered in all-seeing eyes.

I feel as if my eyeballs have enlarged backwards into my head.

From this perspective all sides of her personality are illuminated and there is no 'shadow side'. In a Helium world, no aspect of the persona is shameful, hidden, dirty or ugly. Helium's enlightened ability to illuminate the naked soul contrasts with our terrestrial life in which the soul enters the body. Trapped inside a dense and solid skull with two holes for eyes, only the front of our brain receives light. Seeking to follow this light, our awareness migrates towards the eyes, splitting our illuminated, frontal consciousness from our posterior and shady subconscious. Until we return to the central, vertical axis, part of our being will forever remain hidden in shadow. Henceforth this shadow side will only emerge in deliria, dreams, delusions, sexual fantasies and fears, when daylight floods our night.

Take a moment to notice where your personal awareness is located in your body. For most of us it is at a point in front of our eyes. We imagine that this is where we live. This one-sided consciousness creates a world of division. Now splits into then, creating past and future. Here splits into there, creating territory. Love splits from hate, good splits from bad, light from dark. We develop preferences, and these preferences consolidate into an identity. Our patients express this in sentences such as "I love the sun and I hate the cold" "I love money and I fear poverty" "I am a democrat" "I am an atheist" etc. This one-sided identification is shadowed by a feeling of disease and despair, the inability the achieve wholeness. Welcome to the wonderful world of psora.

Returning to the original words of the proving:

Dark feeling coming down on me. Sadness, feeling **unwell.** Like a **shadow sinking down from above and behind.** Strong desire to kneel down by the bed, **stretch out** my upper body on the bed and pray (which I did). I wish somebody would come and take care of me. I want to be **carried away, out of this dimension and into another one.** I want to **fly away.** I feel **trapped** inside this confused **head,** which is aching. I want my **old head** back. I am crying, more when thinking of the symptoms, realising that I might be trapped inside this head for a long time. I wish I could **curl up** in bed, hide under the covers and sleep for years – to get away. I think **nobody is hearing my prayer.**

Not enjoying the now. Not connecting as parting was so painful, **over-shadowing** the now.

Feeling as if I was born again as the terrible process has become clear.

I feel like I am dancing very close to **my shadow,** very smoothly and in harmony with it. It feels like **my shadow** now. I feel more at one with it and with myself. I suppose its resonance must be **slightly above me** for me to be aware of it, even though it is now very close to me, **like my shadow.**

I feel like I am filled with **black** treacle and it is getting more and more difficult to move and see clearly.

Lately, I have been drawn to buying and wearing **black clothes** which is very unusual for me. Black is the one 'colour' I cannot bear wearing and always gives me the feeling that it stops anything going in or out – that it blocks completely.

Sensation of something **black** grabbing hold of the back of my neck and the back of my head.

I feel wretched and **black**, about myself and my life. I feel isolated, blocked, wretched about my abilities and myself.

Chilliness after a strong, **dark feeling came down on me**. I wanted to **curl up** in bed, hide under the covers and sleep for years.

Chilly after crying, with a sad, **black feeling**.

This psoric shadow is not only individual but global, as psora is a collective ailment.

Have a real sense of something impending, that something is going to happen this week. As if on a psychic level, a certain vibrational pattern is dying or disintegrating and is going to allow another calamity to unleash itself on the world: **darkness**, obliteration, destruction, the calm before the storm, change, unnatural quietness.

As long as Helium is positioned directly above the vertex, vertically aligned with the universal axis of truth, they perceive a holistic and enlightened picture of the self and the world, perceiving all sides of the persona in the bright light of love. It is only when they enter the body and misalign themselves into the there and then, front and back, light and shadow that the painful psoric process of life begins. While Hydrogen teaches us about the separation from God and collective psora, Helium teaches us about the first stage of slipping into individual psora, with all its shadowy results. In this context it is worth noting that Helium also displays a strong affinity to itchy skin.

> Tao is obscured when men understand only one pair of opposites or concentrate only on a partial aspect of being.
>
> Then clear expression also becomes muddled by mere wordplay, affirming this one aspect and denying all the rest.
>
> What use is this struggle to set up "No" against "Yes", and "Yes" against "No"?
>
> Better to abandon this hopeless effort and seek true light!
>
> There is nothing that cannot be seen from the standpoint of the "Not-I".

And there is nothing which cannot be seen from the standpoint of the "I".

If I begin by looking at anything from the viewpoint of the "Not-I", then I do not really see it, since it is "Not-I" that sees it.

If I begin from where I am and see it as I see it, then it may also become possible for me to see it as another sees it.

Hence the theory of reversal that opposites produce each other, depend on each other, and complement each other.

However this may be, life is followed by death; death is followed by life.

The possible becomes impossible; the impossible becomes possible.

Right turns into wrong and wrong into right – the flow of life alters circumstances and thus things themselves are altered in their turn.

But disputants continue to affirm and deny the same things they have always affirmed and denied, ignoring the new aspects of reality presented by the change in conditions.

The wise man therefore, instead of trying to prove this or that point by logical disputation, sees all things in the light of direct intuition.

He is not imprisoned by the limitations of the "I", for the viewpoint of direct intuition is that of both "I" and "Not-I".

Hence he sees that on both sides of every argument there is both right and wrong.

He also sees that in the end they are reducible to the same thing, once they are related to the pivot of the Tao.

The pivot of Tao passes through the centre where all affirmations and denials converge.

He who grasps the pivot is at the still-point from which all movements and oppositions can be seen in their right relationship.

Abandoning all thought of imposing a limit or taking sides, he rests in direct intuition.

Chuang-Tzu[2]

References

1   Lao-Tsu. *Tao Te Ching* (Feng G-F, English J, Lippe T. trans.) New York NY: Vintage Books; 1989. Chapter 23 Available as Kindle edition and also online at: www.questia.com/Online Library
2   Chuang-Tzu The Pivot. In: Merton T (ed) *The Way of Chuang-Tzu*. New York NY: New Directions; 1965.

5

HELIUM CM COLLECTIVE SPIRITUALITY

The most beautiful experience we can have is the mysterious – the fundamental emotion which stands at the cradle of true art and true science.

Albert Einstein[1]

No matter how profound one's understanding may be, there is always a deeper level. Helium CM is based on a proving conducted by Silvie Gowen. I call Silvie the 'magic prover' because of her amazing ability to listen to whispers. Some information from other provers in her proving group is included. Truly a magic 'proving group'.

While many of the themes appear in previous sections, Silvie's proving takes them to the next potency of perception. Note the similarities between the different proving accounts and remember that this proving was undertaken by many people in different countries who had no knowledge of what they were proving.

I have divided Silvie's proving into two parts: Helium CM and Helium MM. The first part, which consists mainly of selected proving symptoms, reflects the soul's journey from spirit into matter as described in the chapter Helium 10M. The second part, Helium MM, gives us a glimpse into the genetics of incarnation, the complex pathway from singularity to diversity.

It is important to realise that I have arranged the themes and the sequence of the proving to reflect my own understanding. Proving symptoms are not given in chronological order, so you will need to refer to the full proving for the original sequence. While many symptoms have been left out, others represent more than one topic and have been duplicated.

Helium CM begins with separation from all-embracing universal love, light and sound, and ends with pregnancy and birth, with all the pain and isolation that result from life in a physical body. Throughout this proving we can clearly recognise the stages detailed in Dr Newton's account of the soul's journey: the lessons of karma, group meetings and pacts, choosing a purpose for the next lifetime, leaving the 'school' and finally entering the physical body. Most significant of all from a clinical point of view is the stage of hovering between worlds with a strong reluctance to occupy a physical body.

The reason for this reluctance is the painful separation from divine love, combined with the perception that the material world is an impure and contaminated place that is full of lies. The need to survive is the source of all lies, but to the Helium patient, truth is more important than survival.

We begin the journey with the endless love of the divine universal soul. This pure energy is symbolised by the light and warmth of a thousand suns. It also manifests as sound, as at source all energies are one. At this point Helium touches Hydrogen and from here the painful parting must take place.

Leaving the One

Universal love

I woke feeling universally loved. I felt very loved by the world yet not on an individual level.

In my inner vision I saw a pow-wow ending in a sun dance. It was about gathering unity rather than separation, a sensation of quickening inside and the gathering of like minds, universal consciousness.

I felt I was witnessing, like watching a game of chess. It was all about love freeing and not binding, the spirit was animating and activating.

Love becomes the inner motive for our actions. Strongest manifestation of the power of the spirit.

As an individual, you make your choice and then you become part of the whole and lose your individuality.

It's like I had forgotten what this was about, to connect to the experience of the One. Like knowing, yet not experiencing it through the senses.

The divine

Dream of waiting for the lift (also waiting for light) to the sixth or seventh floor to meet our Father.

The seventh floor would represent the period of hydrogen and helium if we started counting from the radioactive base.

I felt there was still a divine connection, not needing human company. Or was I not recognising man as the manifestation of the divine.

Sun

Why so warm? I have newly come from the sun.

Do I not receive, not reflect or not retain? All a dream, will I rejoin the sun?

Light

The light I was seeing was brighter than I had ever seen before.

I felt it was all about returning to the force of light, and with that I kept seeing halos and auras, like everything was joined together and was all light, everything merged and no space in between.

The periodic table and specifically the seven noble gases offer an interesting correspondence with the seven days of creation in the Bible. We can note the analogy between the heavenly light of Helium and the first day of creation in the Bible.

The first day represents the evolution from formless void (Hydrogen) to spiritual light (Helium). What is interesting is the nature of this light. Since God didn't create the sun and the moon until the fourth day (Krypton), this is not the light of the sun that we can see. It is the hidden light of infinity, the spiritual light of God.

> In the beginning, God created the heavens and the earth.
> The earth was without form and void, and darkness was over the face of the deep.
> And the Spirit of God was hovering over the face of the waters.
> And God said, "Let there be light", and there was light.
> And God saw that the light was good.
> And God separated the light from the darkness.
> God called the light Day, and the darkness he called Night.
> And there was evening and there was morning, the first day.

Sound

On the swirling margins of the void, light and sound are merged into one energy from which the world was created.

The sounds I was hearing were fitting the light I was seeing.

Dream of being at a concert and being really cheered up by the music. During the music I was given sheets of wax to make candles with. I felt they were made out of sound and I was told they were beautiful movement.

Thoughts of the story of the Wizard of Oz when the scarecrow was taken off the pole. No brain, no heart, minus courage and thoughts of the development of brain, heart and spinal cord, but with the cord I had written chord, and I heard each organ as if I was hearing their creation. Like I could hear the sound of the organs.

Between the worlds

Beginning the journey

I was on my way to diversity and back.

Dream: In a departure lounge cocooned from the outside world between flights, in transit, neither here nor there.

I felt only half here yet functioning very well. I felt clear, efficient, light and calm, as if I had left my other half in a dream.

Feels as if I'm on the edge all the time, not a precipice.

Am I awake during sleep and asleep during waking?

Entering the maze

Seeing the shape of a maze in my inner vision. A spiral maze. The spiral of the self and the search for self, symbolising the wandering of the soul circling inward and outward, seeking nourishment and experience from the outside and from within itself to finally achieve its goal of enlightenment.

I could hear, "All you do is leave a secure thread of light on the path before re-entering the maze."

Then I have an image of spiralling downwards through lilacs and mauves and white vibration. As I do, I pass through many flashes of other lives and experiences that I am simultaneously living and passing through to get to this point of birth, this point of incarnation. And here I will stop for a 'time' (and how illusory is time?!) before I pass onwards in my soul's journey.

I was staying at some sort of huge conference centre with our usual holiday group. We were sitting round deciding what to do and what to wear. The entrance doorway was different to how it would normally be and I could not work out how to get through it and out. Then every time I did go through it, I came out a different way, and went through different corridors – a bit like a maze really.

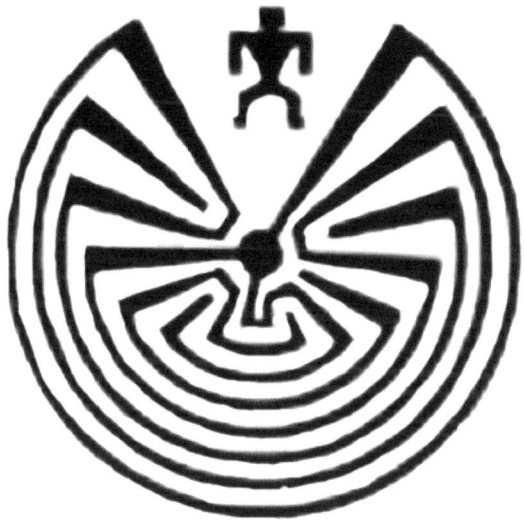

Figure 5.1 *The man in the maze, an emblem of the Tohono O'odham Nation*

The labyrinth is an archetypal symbol found in many ancient traditions. Researchers have come across the use of labyrinths as part of ceremonial journeys in ancient Egypt. The labyrinth represents the soul's journey into the physical world. They are also mentioned in the Bible as well as in the Cabbala.[i]

All life moves in spiral form: From the microcosm of our DNA to the macrocosm of the spiralling galaxies of deep space. The spiral appears in our fingerprints and in the whorl of our crown (vertex, vortex), as well as in nature in the form of shells, flowers and whirlpools. It is a symbol of growth and evolution, a metaphor for the enfolding of spirit into matter and the unfolding of matter returning to spirit.

The labyrinth is a pattern with one single path. There are no tricks and no dead ends. This symbol is employed to represent a person's journey through life. Unlike a maze, which has more than one path and forces choice and confusion, the labyrinth has a single path that meanders into the centre and then guides the traveller safely out again.[2]

---

[i] Throughout the text I have spelt the word Cabbala in this way. There are several different spellings for this word, each signifying different traditions and esoteric thoughts. Personally I prefer the initial letter C to K or Q, as it's vessel shape depicts the receptive (The literal meaning of the word Cabbala is 'to receive' or 'the receptive'). The distinction between K and C will become clear in the study of Krypton. Nevertheless it should be stated that the Hebrew spelling of the word begins with the letter Quoph ('Coof'), which is more akin to K.

It is important to emphasise that the word maze is used more frequently than labyrinth in the proving. To qualify as a maze, a design must have choices in the pathway, indicating that the soul has many options during its decent.

Figure 5.1 originates from the Papago Indians of southern Arizona and depicts a man exiting a labyrinth, and is most often seen in basketry and occasionally in Hopi silver art. Labyrinths are common motifs in ancient Native American rock art and often resemble those found in ancient Greece and other parts of the world.

The labyrinth is used as a tool for healing, meditation and for settling the mind. Walking the labyrinth allows the meditator to focus his thoughts and to gain to insight into his life. It provides the opportunity to re-envision goals, make decisions and evaluate his progress.

Figure 5.2 shows the beautifully preserved pavement labyrinth at Chartres Cathedral, dating from the 13th century.

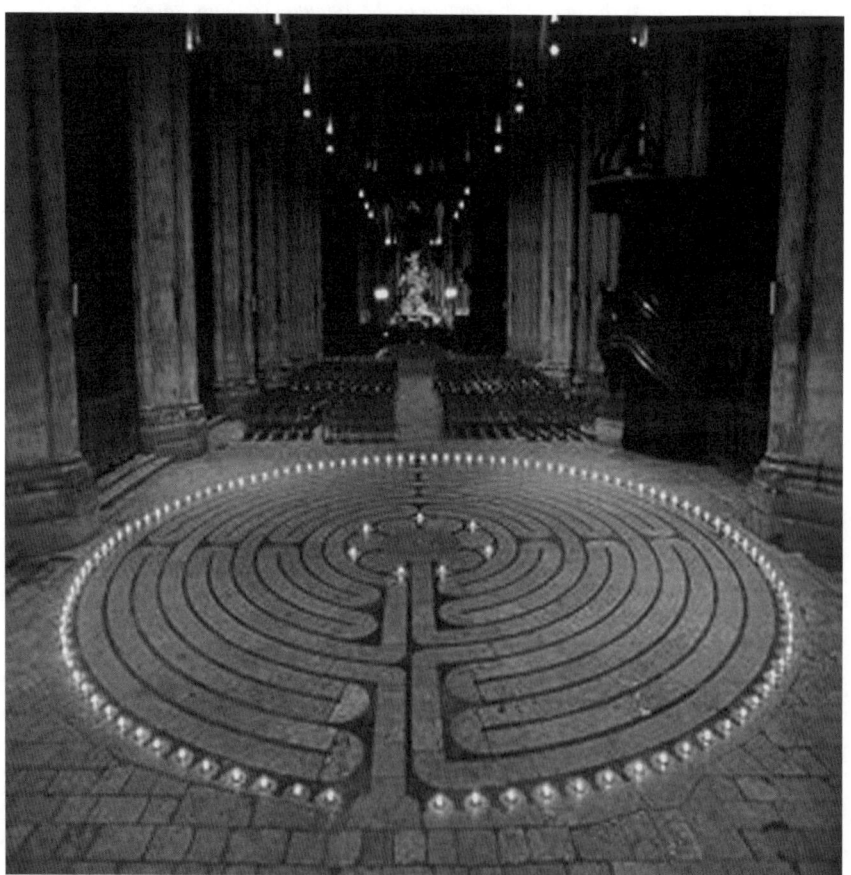

Figure 5.2 *The Chartres Cathedral Labyrinth*

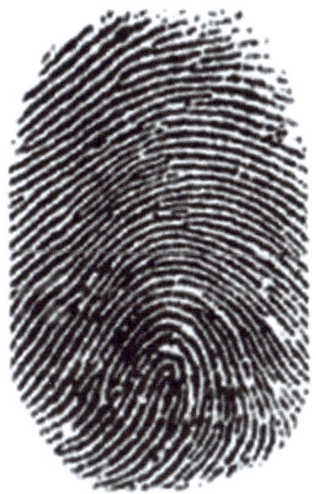

Figure 5.3 A thumbprint whorl

Figure 5.3 shows an image of a thumbprint whorl. Note its similarity to a labyrinth.

This spiral line represents the unification of male (line, light) and female (void, circle) energy, which is the Helium moment of conception and incarnation.

The labyrinth theme also appears in the proving as an image of a thumbprint, our individual signature of existence and arguably a blueprint for our unique journey through the maze.

I had an inner vision of my thumbprint and then I saw beautiful labyrinths and maze patterns. I realised the thumbprint I saw was mine and familiar.

The hum of Helium
Imprint of thumb
Will thy will be done?

It is interesting to see that some schools of palmistry relate the fingerprint to the purpose and journey of the soul. In his book *LifePrints*, hand analyst Richard Unger teaches a method of decoding people's life mission by interpreting their fingerprints.[3]

Reluctance to incarnate

Sadness at having to be born again, sad leaving where I had come from.

Not connecting as parting is so painful.

Sensation of being very immature, not yet ready to be in this world.

It felt like my soul is reluctant to inhabit a body – a reluctance.

I was not sure whether I wanted to join in with life.

Sensation like a shocked foetus leaving the oneness. By not being fully in the body, it reduces the pain of disconnection, disconnected from love.

I don't feel ready for the world yet, unsure in actions what to do next. People were demanding attention which I could give, but what was their panic?

I'm putting things off all the time. The word 'resistant' came up, wasting opportunities.

Remembering previous states, heavenly. Feeling of not wanting to go and do it again, just wanting to be. I was trying to deny that I existed.

I dreamt I was changing my mind about catching the train because I was unsure whether it was the right one. I pushed a small baby through the window before climbing onto the moving train.

I hear people telling me how good life is but I'm not willing to experience it. I feel like a butterfly with closed wings.

Head very cool, desire the sun to warm and soften. No impulse to engage in life.

Knocking on door, didn't go to open it.

I felt I was locked out of my own home.

Dream of keys broken in locks.

Not pure enough

It felt as if the world was not pure enough.

Too open an impression to all possibilities so I have to withdraw. Feel delicate so create gross. Too much impurity.

Truth

I didn't want to be lied to anymore.

I feel I have no true friends, no one is speaking the truth.

I felt I was believing none of what I hear and only half of what I see.

Felt that truth shattered the bonds of separation. It felt we were never given more than we were ready for.

This is about giving birth to self and truth.

I felt unsure. I only wanted to write truth not duality and I was not sure I wanted to join in with life.

We (humans) certainly don't see the same thing.

Better not to reveal than not speak the truth.

I desperately desired contact but I didn't know how. Rather no contact than to be lied to.

Only animals' contact with man causes lying.

Not leaving a mark

I found it hard to put any mark on paper at all.

I was pressing my face into the sofa but I didn't want to leave a mark so others would know what I had been doing. Sensation of not wanting to leave an impression or mark of where I have been.

It feels like a mark on the sand waiting for the tide to come in and obliterate it.

I feel like an empty page, not a written but an embossed page. So do I see and do the reverse?

The blank page seems open to any impression but it also feels like a closed book. Closed but open – opposites.

Unable to tell what temperature I am. I'm trying to deny I exist.

Delusion I kept seeing cut-off trails of creatures in the snow as if they weren't there anymore.

Groups and lessons

Karma

As if I had dreamt I had done it all before.

Learning

Seeing the shape of a maze in my inner vision. A spiral maze. The spiral of the self and the search for self, symbolising the wandering of the soul circling inward and outward, seeking nourishment and experience from the outside and from within itself to finally achieve its goal of enlightenment. Your spiralling dance through life also turns you outward, linking you with others through the group soul or collective unconscious that pervades and encompasses all life. You have a part to play assisting in the spiritual journey of others as they also do in yours.

Remembering and not wanting to repeat mistakes. Only fully loving if giving and receiving.

It was like you didn't have to remember. Things were automatic and you could relearn the rest.

Maybe the withdrawing was the thought that you had nothing to contribute to the world. The best teaching is by example. I felt like everyone was going around saying "I have this right" without the responsibility that goes with it.

Game of life

Felt I didn't understand the rules of life – the game of life.

I wasn't sure whether I was here or just observing, not part of the game of life.

Forgotten the ways of the world.

Purpose of the game

It was like I was observing the games and I thought who made up the rules? It felt like everybody forgot the game because they were so absorbed that they forgot their purpose. It felt easier to withdraw than to trust my senses.

On waking there was a shock realising my destiny. I wasn't sure if I was in the right time or right body. Even though I didn't feel ready, I couldn't put it off any longer.

Being well brings total responsibility.

Honouring other paths, as all paths are sacred.

Friends, groups, pacts

Am I a foetus about to change its mind? It was all about honouring pacts made previously and the doubt was would others remember? I felt I could honour my side but would others remember?

Question: Was I ready to honour the pact I had made in a previous lifetime?

Dream: Driving up a hill in a left-hand drive car. A friend with their son and younger daughter were in the back. It was very cold and windy, so I drove them right up to the school and we had to be silent. I was by the son and there was a desire to be kissed by the father who wasn't there. The feeling was that if I didn't make contact, there wouldn't be any parting.

Connection and disconnection

Disconnected

Extremely internalised, like I was very still and gazing out at the world, not really connecting.

I felt I couldn't discern or discriminate, so I wasn't letting anything in.

Desire to sleep to forget lack of connection.

I felt I was sick due to not being able to connect in case the contact wasn't returned.

I felt like dancing alone. Felt the separation was the greatest pain imaginable. No connection in our own world.

No sleep, no leaving the body, no reprieve, ever more inwards, but it felt I needed to persevere and reverse the process. If I'm not needed here I would prefer to be somewhere else (depression). It felt like partial contact was too painful yet when I did connect with people it felt very light and bright.

Isolation

Felt like we had much to share even though the path was solitary.

Withdrawn emotionally, so much pain. Close off the outside world and retreat.

We come in and go out alone.

Lack of intimacy. Easier to withdraw than be rejected.

Re-connecting on earth

The rift between people felt painful. The man in the dream was the one to connect with. Sensation of not wanting to leave an impression or mark of where I have been. Felt like a permanent déjà vu feeling.

I looked across and saw a man un-partnered; he started walking around towards me. I was waiting outside the dances for him to come. We would have to connect.

Dream: At last I reconnected with my lover.

I felt a need to act not just to think, do I have to imagine it first? I knew I had to make contact, a very passive state.

Opposite of what I had been feeling. I feel like everyone is a potential friend. Passive with potential but no action yet.

Arrival

Intention and action

I need to create rather than passively observe. Time for action really.

It feels as if I have more thoughts and less instincts.

I felt a need to act not just to think, do I have to imagine it first? I knew I had to make contact, a very passive state.

Never feeling like I'm quite ready, it feels like the 'how' is missing.

No dependence on others with which to formulate ideas. No interaction, just internal action.

On waking I wrote "expectant state more fulfilling than the action" or "totally fulfilled after the action". The sensation was like being warmed by the light.

Delusion as if I have done something active, the thoughts were so vivid I thought I had done it.

Usually the thought is just enough and there is no need to express it. It felt the dream needed to be created and the words began with M: manifest, manifold, magnanimous, etc.

Sensation I'm putting things off all the time. The word 'resistant' came up, wasting opportunities.

Sacrifice limitation through action.

The key broke in the lock and the lock was broken and there were two parts of the key and there was no turning and no action.

Pregnancy

In my inner vision I kept seeing a placenta and it looked as if it was hanging from a tree.

There was an issue on the radio about foetuses not feeling pain. I thought they don't scar but it's not that they don't feel pain, both physical and mental (soul enters foetus when it is fully developed, perhaps between 12 and 14 weeks). Don't be deluded that foetuses don't feel pain.

I felt the shock of first breath.

Thoughts of emeralds.

Egyptians believed that emeralds stood for rebirth and fertility and could ease the pains of childbirth.[4]

Dream of snuffly babies. The worse thing about it was they could not let the air in, they couldn't smell their mother. It was a good time to heal as a foetus as it wouldn't cause scarring.

Coming and going

Dr Newton writes that at this early stage the soul can freely enter and leave the foetus's body or even move from one womb to another:

Dreamt that I was going to give birth to another woman's baby but it wasn't clear: Was it me who was pregnant and me who was going to give her the baby after the birth? Or was it her that was pregnant and her that was going to have the baby? If I was pregnant, had there been a semen implantation? I was very puzzled by all this in the dream.

Where am I? Am I in the right bed or womb? Not sure if I'm in the right womb, is this what I really need? Fulfilling destiny, second thoughts.

Entering the head

I had other delusions that I had a large head covered in all-seeing eyes.

Dream: My mother showed me a model of a much smaller skull. The question I asked was, "What did they put in the water that year?"

Dream a man with double jaws, a smaller one within the larger.

Birth

I was in some Japanese-inspired surroundings. An egg-shaped pond with ice-cold water, and a thin layer of ice on top. I didn't know if it was muddy or full of plants, fishes, other creatures or anything dangerous. I undressed completely and jumped in after a short hesitation. The others around thought it was a great, impressive, respectful thing to do. My body broke the ice as I jumped into the pool. The water was ice-cold but clear. I went all the way to the bottom and then rose slowly upwards. The sun was shining through the water making all the bubbles glitter. I had to take a deep breath while still under water and found that I could breathe in the water. When I broke through the top it was like going through a membrane. I rose from the pond feeling like a new person, a cleaned person, actually more 'me' than ever. I was in contact with all of myself, and felt very whole. It felt like an initiation and I was met with deep respect afterwards.

References

1   Einstein A. Essay – The World As I See It. In: Seelig C (ed.), *Ideas and Opinions, based on Mein Weltbild*, New York NY: Bonzana Books; 1954, pp. 8–11. An abridged version is available online at http://tinyurl.com/8gaj4.

2   Saward J. *Mazes or Labyrinths, What's the difference and what types are there?* Labyrinths and Mazes Resource Centre Photo Library and Archive. Available online at http://tinyurl.com/8649exp.

3   R. Unger R. *Lifeprints: Deciphering Your Life Purpose from Your Fingerprints*. Berkeley CA: Crossing Press; 2007.

4   Emerald accelerates birth-giving in Ancient Egypt The *First Egyptian Arabic English Tourist Newspaper*. Available online at: http://tinyurl.com/6tzpuf7.

6

MEDITATION PROVING OF HELIUM

Please skip this section if you feel uncomfortable with meditation provings, as I once did. The following is what I have called a Mini Meditation proving. I have done my share of full Hahnemannian provings and will continue to do them. But alongside these classical provings, I have experimented with parallel Mini Meditation provings, checking and rechecking their accuracy. These provings often expose another facet or configuration of the remedy picture. Provings, however conducted, are only suggestions for materia medica. I have found that there is a definite advantage to doing a Mini Meditation proving with a highly sensitive person. Speed and an unusual perspective are two of these advantages. It is however essential that the prover be blind to the remedy.

My test for the authenticity of these meditation provings has been twofold. Firstly, while the meditation provers did not know the remedy, the theme of the pictures produced should reflect the totality and essence of the conventional proving. Secondly, their effectiveness in the clinic: Do prescriptions based on these pictures actually work? I have repeatedly proved the validity my wife's meditation provings in the clinic.

My wife Camilla has participated in fifteen Hahnemannian provings and edited several more. She has developed the sensitivity and acuity of senses to produce excellent Mini Meditation provings. She is quite clairvoyant and born to a line of psychically sensitive people. Her Mini Meditation provings are unexpected, vivid and accurate. I particularly appreciate how she often illuminates a more 'negative' side of the remedy, one that often matches real suffering.

In this proving the remedy was only held but not taken. Camilla had no idea what the remedy was. Like me she had a very different image of Helium and was highly surprised to find out what the remedy was. Yet it made sense.

You may be of the scientific branch of homeopathy and consider meditation provings an abomination. I respect that. Remember, you are invited to ignore this section and save yourself the indignation. Take it or leave it, what you don't know won't hurt you.

The proving was recorded verbatim from the moment it begun.

Helium Mini Meditation proving

Observation: Moving her head and neck back and forth.

I feel as if my neck and throat are swelling like a goitre, like a bullfrog.

I feel like a fat loser, a computer nerd who sits in a dark room, swollen and fat. A hacker who sits by a computer all day and doesn't get out and smell the fresh air, who sits in the dark, dirty room, disgusting and oozing, yuck.

Like a fat wanker with a goitre. Lonely and misanthropic, who doesn't want to see people.

Tingling in my scalp on the left side.

I feel a big great swelling in my external throat.

But there is something righteous, a brilliance of the mind, a knowing that is there. The mind is sharper than most people's, very sharp. But the mind and the body are not in synch. The mind is brilliant but the body is gross, swollen and fat and with a goitre. The mind is razor-sharp regarding computers and hacking, like the guy in 'Girl with the dragon tattoo'. Filthy, with a gross apartment full of dirt and shit, but a genius. Never had a shower. A big discrepancy between the mind and the body. In most people things average out so you don't have that big a discrepancy. Here there is a huge difference. The cut of point is the throat. Fat and physical decay.

But the mind is brilliant: fast, accurate, making millions of connections like a computer. Understanding them and making the most of them because the mind is like a computer but more creative. Living off fast food, pizza and coke. The brilliance of the mind is limited, applies to computers but not to emotional intelligence, diet or exercise. A solitary person, no friends or hobbies, doesn't want to see people, never leaving the house. Everything is virtual. A very one-sided person. Maybe he experienced trauma in the past, in childhood, like sexual abuse, seeing something violent, something that would make you cut off. A lot of fears underneath that are suppressed, he is not even aware of them. Claustrophobia, fear of lots of people in one place. No friends, no boyfriends or girlfriends. Maybe a sexual perversion that is suppressed, even a serial killer, not that they necessarily would, but they could be. Maybe a suppressed violence, but I don't feel the violence. A single-minded and partial personality. Like some aspect of the personality has not been able to develop, the sexual and the identity, who you are, no reference points. Trauma or abuse that dwarfs one's development. He does not develop into a healthy adult personality or a clear sexual identity. Social antipathy and lack of contact, all the contact is virtual, so he could go mental (crazy-JS). A lot of suppression. But there is no anger or violence, just a curiosity of how other humans would think or feel under pressure. It is as if this persona's humanity is missing, not a well-rounded person with grief, joy, anger or happiness. If he would extend to serial killing, it would come from a curiosity about how humans would react in extreme danger, experimenting to try and under-stand how humans function. Like an alien with some human qualities but not the full range and a scientific, clinical curiosity, not from emotions. A lack of empathy. This person could not put themselves in another person's shoes, lacking empathy, a one-sided case. A huge loneliness but without the emotion, this person doesn't feel lonely. Isolation with virtual contact, computer, chat rooms, all virtual. He wouldn't be able to understand. Like a kid who pulls the wings off a fly, not malicious, just curiosity. Unfeeling but not really cruel. But a brilliant single mindedness regarding the computer aspect of it. Could relate to Nazis doing experiments on twins, to see how much pressure a human being can take. How high can they fly with an airplane before they pop, or how deep can they go in a submarine. The morality of using humans as guinea pigs doesn't enter the equation, like the part of the brain with empathy and sympathy is not there. Almost not a crime because it's not perceived as a crime. Something is not there to perceive that what I am doing is sick. In court they would say, "Yes, but we needed to find out". They don't care about individual humans suffering, they would say, "We are doing this for humanity, the greater good, all of humanity will benefit and fuck the individual", no sympathy for the indi-vidual. It would be easy to brainwash this person to become a one-cause recruit. They don't understand the individual. They are interested in the collective in an analytical way, a project or a job. But they don't really care about humanity. Interested in the riddle or the mystery, intellectual knowl-edge and facts. Missing humanity, empathy and love feelings. Bad stuff suppressed in the background, neglect or abuse that has totally killed the human side, that which makes us human, but they are unaware of it. This is an awful place to be but they don't even know that they are there so it doesn't matter too much. To them it is normal. Lack of ability to look at the self objectively. They would not be able to see that it is missing, can't see what they lack in love and friends. They look at us and think: What is all that love bullshit? They probably feel lucky that they are not part of it. Very detached, a detached observer. Like looking from a third person viewpoint, like it's not me I'm talking about. Maybe a schizophrenic, someone with Asberger's, like another persona. I feel detached from it but I can understand it. Moral values and ethics are not congruous to them; they don't see it like that at all. If you put them in court and prison for 25 years they would not comprehend what they have done wrong. There is no joy, no feeling, but they don't know they don't have it. Detached and indifferent.

It feels like there is swelling and fluid retention.

I have since verified much of this picture in practice, including the ailments from sexual abuse. This proving feels very different to the previous picture. The basic themes however are similar. It is not difficult to imagine how detached Helium could deteriorate into such a configuration. The separation between head and body, obesity, dirt, detachment from the physical, indifference and apathy are all common themes. It is not sufficient to study the light. We must delve into the shadows.

The image I have is of a bird in a gilded cage, like in Nazi concentration camps. I feel like I am a prisoner kept in a cell with bars on it. I have some use to the Nazis, they keep me alive because I am useful to them. That is the only thing that saves my life and keeps me alive. I am aware of life going on around me. I hear of terrible atrocities, world developments, etc. but they are all outside of me. I am aware of it, but not able to participate. I am of use to the Nazis, but not of value.

From Prover 40

It might be interesting to compare the last symptom to the related remedy Bald Eagle (Haliaeethus Leucocephalus). As in the Helium proving it depicts two suns, but in Haliaeethus the second is a dark or black sun. Haliaeethus brings forth images of the Hitler and Natsism. The black sun and the eagle are symbols of the Nazi regime.[1]

Reference

1   Black Sun (occult symbol). Wikepedia. See: http://tinyurl.com/cregs5 and http://tinyurl.com/8367kyl
Also see Nemesis (hypothetical star) at http://tinyurl.com/8367kyl

7

HELIUM SYNTHESIS

The following offers a synthesis of Helium, based on sensations and functions or the 'verb' of this remedy. For more information on this method of synthesis, please see *The Dynamic Materia Medica-Syphilis*.[1] Please note that sensation and function are interchangeable and form a cycle, so you can read them in reverse order as well. In other words, one could alternatively read "sensation: fused, function: separate".

Sensation: separated
Function: Fuse

Sensation: Dark
Function: Create light

Sensation: Leaving the one
Function: Create a new one

Sensation: Floating and observing from above
Function: Must manifest on earth

Sensation: Upright and above. Cannot lean forward into life.
Function: Lean forward into action

Adjectives: Light, dark, shadow, ethereal, heavy, fat, inert, action, potential, plan, manifest, disconnected

Nouns: Soul, body, sun, eagle, healing, music, meditation, prayer, purpose, mission, shadowless, shadow, clean, dirty

Image: Reluctance of the soul to enter the dirty, dangerous material world. To act or not to act, and for what purpose?

Chakra: Crown[i]

---

[i] The crown chakra is violet in colour and is located at the top of the head. It is the chakra of divine purpose and destiny. This chakra is said to be your own place of connection to God. When unbalanced, you may experience depression, lack of grounding and lack of inspiration (because you are disconnected from your spiritual source).

Day of creation: First day

Alchemical stage: Calcination

Colour: Violet

Musical scale: B

Whammy: Spirituality

Location: The poles

Time: The solstices

Books

The Holy Zohar (Cabbala),[3] *Sefer Yetzirah,*[4] *The World to Come* by Dara Horn[5]
These are just a few selected samples, there are many more volumes coming
from a variety of esoteric traditions.

References

1   Sherr J. *The Dynamic Materia Medica – Syphilis.* 2nd edition, Glasgow: Saltire
    Books; 2013.
2   Berg Y, bar Yocak S. *The Holy Zohar: The Book of Abraham.* Toronto ON: Research
    Centre of Kabbalah; 2001.
3   Matt DC (trans). *Zohar: Pritzker Edition* (6 vols. to date). Stanford CA: Stanford
    University Press; 2004–2011.
    For more translations see: https://en.wikipedia.org/wiki/Zohar
4   Kaplan A (ed & trans). *Sefer Yetzirah, The book of creation in theory and practice.*
    York Beach MA: Samuel Weiser; 1990.
5   Horn D. *The World to Come.* New York NY: WW Norton & Co Inc; 2006.

8

HELIUM CASES

I have collected cases from as many sources as possible to show different approaches and aspects of the remedy. I have presented the cases as given to me, and other then slight grammatical editing they remain so.

Some of the follow ups are long and others short. This makes no difference to me in the context of learning about the remedy. I do not subscribe to the notion that one needs years of good follow ups to learn something about a particular remedy. Sometimes a remedy will be highly curative in a short time, thus dealing with the relevant issues before moving on to other remedies. This is in accordance with the *Organon*, and in some situations may indicate a more profound action of the remedy, as it cures the deepest underlying susceptibility. What is important is not the length of reaction but the quality of the cure. Every case in which the remedy acts on the patients can be instructive, so long as one can differentiate between different levels of cure or even accidental provings.

CASE 8.1 'Fear of birth and life'

Case from Jeremy Sherr
A female patient, 33 years old, pregnant with her fourth child, two weeks overdue. The midwife wanted to induce her but she refused. Her waters have been broken for four days, but there has been no dilation and contractions have not begun. She was given a few remedies (Caulophyllum, Pulsatilla and others) but with no success. The midwife was beginning to panic. The patient was distressed and contacted me by phone in the middle of the night.

She said, "I've been meditating and in the meditation I saw a Native American Indian man. He said to me that he was the one to be born but he didn't want to be. He said, "It is much easier up here. I can just inflict people with my ideas, I can put thoughts into people's heads and they will write books and music and do things. I don't have to do it myself. It is really hard on earth, I prefer to stay here, I'm scared of birth and of life."

The patient knew then that the baby was reluctant to come.

In another meditation, she saw an eagle. After this meditation, she went for a walk in the forest and she found a feather and a ring lying next to each other.

Rx: Helium 30C

Within one minute of taking the remedy, strong contractions began. In less than an hour a healthy baby was born.

CASE 8.2 'Starry night'

Case from Jeremy Sherr

"I am 36 years old. I have had homeopathic treatment for four years with little improvement. I am very anxious about being here. I couldn't sleep last night. I had a dream that you gave me a 'starry night' remedy. I have been having a tough time with my husband. We have not been sexual for two years. I don't feel dead sexually, I am just not attracted to him. I am passionate and emotional and confused. Should I leave or not – It is a dilemma, how to do what is right for me and not hurt him. The dilemma is also how will it affect my son?

I live in a perfect place. I have a vision of a backyard, wooded and beautiful. Then everything becomes distorted, a cut. And through the cut comes the unconditional love of God. I want unconditional love, but how hard it is to accept it. I need to fall into faith but I have a lot of fear.

I am financially dependent on my husband, how will I live and feel supported? I have a yearning for a total shift in perspective, towards joy and away from fear. I'm all cerebral now, but I want to move from my head to my heart. I want to feel comfortable in my body."

---

[i] This case was originally published in *The American Homeopath* Vol 6 (California, 2000).

Observation: hand moves from head to heart

"I landed in my body and at times I leave it. I want to be totally in it. I started belly dancing, a sensual experience. I love dancing and music. I feel stagnant and when I move I feel better. Internally I am cold, freezing most of the time.

I want to be inspired to reach to the depths of my soul. I feel tired and I've lost inspiration. I am not thirsty, I struggle to drink. I crave sweets.

When I am sad, I shut down completely. It perpetuates my isolation. I don't participate in superficial relationships. I like a relationship to be deep. I isolate myself for self-preservation.

In my dream I was sitting with you and I take the remedy 'starry night'. Then opportunities open up and blossom. I'd like to see things for what they are, but I look at life through a filter. I see great potential in my husband, but he is explosive and has hit me. He is like a baby, throws things and is petty. I want to feel safe.

I have a vision where I'm standing on top of a mountain wearing a white gown. My arms are out. If I just lean forward I would be ok, but I am too afraid to lean into it. I'm too scared to fall into faith. I need to take the fall, to lean forward to follow my dream.

My dream is to be understood and to have a relationship with someone mature. I stand on the mountain, lean forward and fall into the mist on earth. I have so much to take care of on earth. I need to speak my total truth without fear. My basic fear is not being understood by my husband. My husband is a baby, but he says that I am selfish, that I consider myself first and don't nurture him.

My parents divorced when I was six. My mother had severe depression and stayed in bed. I had the consistent feeling of not being understood. Others didn't understand me. People who live in their bodies view life as a journey, they look deeper.

I was poor as a child and thought I would be ok when I had money but I wasn't. Lately I have been taking off my jewellery. I can't wear gold, diamonds, they don't mean anything. I was wearing jewellery to know who I was. I want to be myself. In the past I was being like everyone else. At times I can be out there and be alone.

I have many dreams, vivid ones. I moved to a new place, there was beautiful furniture, a tortoiseshell chair that cost about $10,000. A woman, a part of me, was doing homey things. There was danger, a dangerous man. It was all a façade with violence underneath. I was trying to make it ok. The tortoiseshell was beautiful, so I thought maybe I'll stay.

I had recurring dreams as a child. I am running away from danger and couldn't get anywhere. I am falling, never landing. Going quickly down from a high place, from a four-storey building on a unicycle. I fall on a unicycle and never land.

I have a fear of the dark. I can't watch horror film stuff. Ghosts. I don't want to see spirits, it scares me. I feel spirits, that's ok.

During my mother's pregnancy, her relationship with my father was not good. Her labour was very easy. I flew out of her body.

I have lower back pain when I stand. I like to sit. My neck goes out a lot. I love having it cracked and adjusted.

I feel ovulation pains. I have premenstrual headaches. I hold my breath a lot. It is a conscious effort to take a full body breath.

My hair is grey, I have bags under my eyes. I see my body is aging a lot, it is strange.

A huge thing is I don't lie and I don't like people who lie. No truth could ever be as ugly as a lie unrevealed. Intention is everything."

Rx: Helium 1M

Follow-up 2 months later
"The remedy was working as soon as I left the office. I was standing on the mountain and I knew I needed to take the leap of faith. I even realised that I had seen God already and needed to see the ground beneath my feet.

The remedy was in all the cells of my body. I had realisations about everything, including my relationship with time. I had always been in a battle before, now I don't run out of time. I feel very present.

For the first couple of weeks, I felt a gentle weight on the top of my head, keeping me down. It was comforting and I was present in my body. For the first time I was able to defend myself against my husband and speak up for myself.

I don't have to leave my body anymore. What is so great about leaving my body anyway? I leave my body unattended and open for violation, unless I have a specific intention to leave and safety around it. I am so grateful to be in my body. We are going on vacation and I specified to my husband that anywhere is ok as long as it is at sea level.

I used to have a fear about digging in the ground and putting my hand in the ground. I realise that being close to the earth is hard. My relationship to my body has been one of total discomfort. But going out was leaving it open for violation. Now when I wake up I desire to feel my feet on the ground.

Five days ago I got my period and didn't know it was coming – no PMS. It was a gorgeous, flowing and red period. I enjoyed it, I felt alive.

I am very mindful of doing the laundry, sweeping the floor and being present. The sound of the broom on the floor is pleasurable.

I feel communion and community. I am a part of the community now and to be with people is great.

I am more comfortable in the dark. I slept alone this week with just my son. My husband was away and I felt really comfortable.

My neck and back pain are very good.

After you told me the remedy I had was Helium I remembered that my husband proposed to me in a hot air balloon! What other way to propose to a Helium patient than when her feet are off the ground!

Helium has touched me in my whole being since I was conceived. Am I or aren't I here – do I belong? That is why I needed to be affirmed all the time, to know that I belong. It is nice to have new information now and to be finding a place on earth."

Follow-up 3 and 6 months later
The improvement has continued, doing very well all round. After nine months the issues changed as did the suitable remedies.

Analysis – themes of Helium in this case
The main theme in this case that corresponds to the Helium proving is a soul that does not come completely into the body and is unable to manifest itself fully in life. In the proving there are many themes of mountains in dreams and mental symptoms, with a desire to jump down onto the earth. Correspondingly, there is a feeling of disconnection between the head and the heart, leaving the neck area vulnerable.

A common idea of Helium is of uprightness without the ability to lean away from the vertical. Much faith and courage are required for a soul to take the leap from the vertical into the diagonal turmoil of life. Otherwise the soul will remain forever in a state of static potential, which is neither activated nor manifested. In opposition to these ideas, we see the patient's overly rapid birth. The idea of a vertical line refusing to tilt, and later managing to do so, will become an important factor in our study of dimensions.

The idea of being a baby is also prevalent in Helium. Falling on a unicycle represents the Helium idea of a soul, which is as yet undifferentiated into male and female. Although there is a connection to God's love, it cannot be manifested in a life of physical action. In the patient's dream, the empty tortoiseshell is like a body without a soul.

The idea of 'starry night' as a remedy corresponds to outer space and the realm of the soul. Because of the patient's inability to live a life of action, opportunities do not open up and blossom. It is the same state of unmanifested potential that the patient sees in her husband. In this state a person cannot feel understood because she is not connected via the bodily organs and shell.

Another idea in Helium is the inability to take a full breath, to connect spirit and body. The uprightness of the noble gases is also represented in a sometimes rigid morality. In this case the patient was unable to lie. Her statement that no truth could be as ugly as a hidden lie is simply too noble an idea for life on this earth.

The idea that intention is everything is possibly the ultimate statement of Helium. Intention may be the source of everything but without physical action, it remains unmanifested. The patient's connection to spirits further illustrates the idea of disembodiment. We cannot stand at the peak of the mountain forever. There must be a time to come down into the valley.

CASE 8.3 'Out of body'

Case from Christopher Beaver, USA
A 45 year-old woman who is a professional psychic.

The woman reports, "I have felt out of my body ever since I was a little girl. I enjoy the other world I live in. It is a place where life is kind, sweet and gentle. It has become a problem in the later years of my life. There are just too many times I am not there and not present. I feel like I am hovering and floating out of my body throughout my life. It is the sensation that I am here but not here and I want be here now fully.

My work is not moving forward anymore and I know that it is due to the fact that there is a part of me that does not really care. I know I need to care. I need to care more about the events that are happening in my life and its story. This is the place that I go to when everything gets tough. It is like there is a thin silver cord that connects from me and allows me to go out of my body. I am here and then it is like a zip line out of my body.

This barrier I have has always made me feel safe. I have to say that I feel safe behind this ephemeral wall. It's like gossamer layers on top of each other. I pass through this wall into this amazing, safe place. It feels like everything there is connected and whole. I get a sense of communion there that I often cannot find here. I can see that this is becoming a problem now. I need to be more aware of what I am doing and pay attention or I could start creating serious issues for myself and my family."

Analysis
The basic idea in the case of being here yet not being fully here is creating the sense of incomplete incarnation. The most simple thing we can look at is the patient's language: here/not here, floating and hovering, in and out of the body, the ephemeral wall through which she passes to a safe place where communion is achieved, a zip line out of the body. The basic idea that this is too much takes us to the right side of the periodic table. We can also understand Helium from the idea that they are not fully here on this planet although they are on their way here.

Rx: Helium 1M, dry dose under the tongue

Follow-up 1 month later
"I am here. I feel good. I had a huge emotional collapse for a few days after the remedy. It happened one morning when I woke up, I just felt like all of the ephemeral wall dissolved and flowed into my body. I feel here. There has been an increase in my practice over the last few days which I am happy about, and I can see how I have not had a deep laugh in years. My family and I had a great experience one morning at the kitchen table where I just started laughing and I felt like I had never laughed so hard in all my life. My mood has improved and so has my energy level. The fatigue that I used to feel is now gone. I have more energy than I had before."

Postscript

Continued doses of Helium in various potencies brought about deep emotional and psychological healing for her. The case was finished in 9 months of treatment, which I found interesting because this could represent a birthing cycle. The client continues to do well to this day.

CASE 8.4 'Stuck birth'

Case from Christopher Beaver, USA

A middle-aged female architect whose chief complaint is fibromyalgia.

"The pain is a wandering pain throughout all my body. It travels and floats throughout my whole body. It gives me a sense of wanting to leave, leave my body, leave my life. I have never been here anyway. The pain floats and then gets stuck in a part of my body and there it stays until it floats and travels and gets stuck someplace else.

I am stuck everywhere. Nothing is moving the way I would like it to. My life force is just shot. I have no energy. This feeling of being stuck is literal and metaphorical. I feel like I am just stuck everywhere and even stuck with this body that does not work well either. I hate this. I would like to feel like everything could be fluid again.

I am stuck. It reminds me of birth, as if I am stuck in the birth canal. I cannot come through, there is no breakthrough for me in my life. Stuck like my head is crowned but my body is in that other place. I have been like this all my life now. I want to come out, to come through and be here. Accept my power and be whole, not divided in two. That is why all the pain gets stuck, it's filling in that in between and holding me at this threshold. Can you give me a remedy to break through that wall and be here? This is what I need."

Analysis

The woman had been having homeopathic treatment prior to coming to see me. She had received many polycrest remedies. From her language we can see that this is a clear mineral case as she talks about form, function, flow of energy and finality. It is obvious that there is a strong delusional experience of being stuck in the birth canal, the great in between. This indicates we are dealing with the first and second rows of the periodic table. The fact that the energy is stuck and not flowing, and also that she experiences too much would possibly indicate the right side of the periodic table.

Using Jeremy Sherr's excellent proving of Helium, we can see many of the proving sensations coming through very clearly in the case.

Rx: Helium 1M

Follow-up 1 month later
"I feel as if I have gone through a rebirthing experience. After taking the remedy the pain in my body amplified overnight. I was breathing really hard through the pain as if I was giving birth. My body felt cramped, each muscle felt like it was tightening and releasing through my breathing. The pain was not just pain but a level of ecstasy as well. It was one of those phenomena that hurt and was good and frightening at the same time. After that night I felt better each day, stronger, more encouraged about life. The pain is now 70 percent better. My energy is up as much as that as well. I feel more alive than before. This is the first real sign of hope I have had in a long time."

The patient continued to improve until the pain was 95 percent gone. She would call periodically to update me and she needed several more doses of the remedy over the following five months. This patient continues to refer other patients to me to this day, calling homeopathy the miracle medicine that she always knew it was.

CASE 8.5 'In a cocoon'

Case from Dr Elizabeth Thompson, UK
A 38 year-old woman recovering from breast cancer treatments.

"I am inclined to anaemia and I have a general tiredness, a sense of exhaustion. I have to grapple with things, it gives me anxiety, a panicky feeling, like a pressure, a pressing down. I am responsible, I am totally responsible, completely responsible for nurturing myself. I am on my own."

What is it to be completely responsible?

"It was like they didn't see me, I didn't have any identity. I did have it, but there was a lack of recognition."

What was this like?

"It is a withdrawing energy. I go into my own self-contained world, like a duvet."

Tell me more about this.

"It is safe, cut-off, you cut yourself off from support. Just me, no demands, no one dictating who I am. If I withdraw, I turn help down, they are there, I am here, I am cut-off but I have chosen to cut off. I am over-loved, so I withdraw. I am going into my own world, a retreat, it is safe, I create a cocoon, it is the cotton wool."

What is it like to be present?

"I am stamped on, crushed, I am losing myself. I go into the cocoon. I have to ground myself, I have to be solid, otherwise I will be dispersed into pieces, annihilated. I am not here, I have disappeared. I am pulled apart, tearing me apart, total exposure until there is nothing."

Describe the opposite of nothing.

"There would be a totally expansive sense of self. I would be grounded with a strong sense of who I am and a right to be here. There would be a sense of completion with myself and protection, not containment, a different kind of boundary, more fluid. It is protective like a rubber band, it is stretching, it can expand. The other feeling is much more contraction (*she makes a gesture, which she comes back to, fingers in the centre of the palm*). I have to hold a space where there is no growth, I can't let love in. My father was distant, he cut himself off, there was a disconnection, completely abandoned and lost. It is hard to find myself, the little girl. She needs outside affirmation, there is annihilation, I am not existing, I am not being allowed to exist."

Describe this more.

"I don't feel love, it is cold, I can't feel my own self, there is a disconnection, I am in the void, I don't want to be born, I am wanting to be here, there is nothing to hold on to, nothing to keep me here, it is too hard to be here. I am too sensitive, too vulnerable. I feel different, I shouldn't be here. It is black and nothing, there is no spiritual connection. I have a fear of living and a fear of dying but I can't be in either. I want to be more total, more here and more recognised for who I am."

Analysis

Here we see a key theme of row one of the periodic table: that of existence. We see the vital sensation of the gas with the feeling of not being solid, instead dispersing and expanding. We also get a clear sense of the inner experience of the pain of existence and the need to withdraw into a cocoon. We also see a confirmation of the key issue of the mineral kingdom: to feel complete when one is incomplete.

Rx: My first prescription is **Natrum Nitricum**, but it does not hold. I give her **Helium 200C**.

She emails me in May 2006, five weeks after the remedy.

"I feel a definite shift inside me. I feel calmer and definitely more solid and contented. By solid, I mean more here."

Follow-up in July 2006

Just describe being more solid.

"I am coming in, I could have an impact, I do have knowledge, and I feel more present, more present in my body. As a child I always felt so self-conscious, but now I feel I am here and I don't care, I feel more seen."

CASE 8.6 'Ungrounded mother'

Case from Kåre Troelsen, Denmark

June 2009. A woman aged 28 who has just became a mother. She had already received Natrium Muriarticum form a colleague some years ago which helped her migraines.

So what is happening to you?

"Family, the word, it changed shape after we had our baby P. Since he was born nothing is stable in our lives. I have this monologue in my head because I am alone on parental leave. What does it mean to be parents? How does P. experience us? We lack parental stability like our parents had it (*gesture indicating solid ground*). I would like to give P. the feeling of stability that I had. I have used the last 5 years scrutinising everything about me, forming an opinion about everything. But things have not arrived at the place where they ought to be (*gesture indicating base again*) Health as a basis for our life. We are fighting strong powers, it pulls the carpet away under our feet, what are we supposed to trust? I want to make P. strong and healthy. I miss the ignorance. My mind is working at high speed and under high pressure. I want to give P. the best possible conditions for his development, remove barriers. I am allergic to milk. My mum did not have enough milk, so I was fed buttermilk and vomited blood. I stuttered when I first started to speak and I still do now when I am out of balance.

When I was 6 years old we were in a car accident. My dad died, my mother was brain damaged. I was then alone with mum who was incredibly sad. I feel I have experienced big losses and let-downs in my childhood. I don't have a good relationship to my mother and sister; we live far apart. She is not good on foreign ground, and she has nothing to talk about. My sister is so busy with her family and not inclined to look outside her world. I don't talk to her.

I remember my dreams so clearly! Often I am in an atomic war. I am in a hurry, running, distances are extremely huge. It is very difficult to move in the chaos. Last night I dreamt I was trying to pedal on a scooter and was getting nowhere. In the atomic war I am with a few chosen ones, in a spiritual community, we have knowledge and insight and are trying to communicate it to people, but we have to save ourselves.

I probably don't have the most realistic image of my own body. I've always felt very fat, ugly, I do not want anyone to take photos of me. I always used to look sad on photos. As soon as mirrors are put up and people have an opinion about me, they zoom in on what I don't like. I had anorexia when I was 17–18 years old. It was difficult being a teenager, moving away from home and growing up."

Tell about difficult.

"Losing the safety net, only me. Who am I, what do I want? What do I think? Without a 'business card' (saying this is me), you have to form an opinion about everything. It is only recently that I know what I want. It is a great relief. I am starting to study next year, it is a duty to use your head for something."

Tell me about losing your safety net.

"Am I doing things right? Have I already ruined my baby? Was I not ready to become a mother? What do I do? I am afraid of making a mistake and breaking him. Has the lack of unconditional love in the first two weeks damaged him? Has he lost trust, is he feeling unsafe? No stability, security, trust."

How does that feel?

"It's like I feel the blood leaving my head and going to my body. To be a human being is suddenly not a concrete thing. Losing your identity as a human being, becoming a creature, being in the world. I feel guilty every time I turn on the TV. I won't eat anything that is not organic. I feel like a stone age person in the space age. Too many questions, my head can't contain it all. I feel I can't take on the full responsibility."

You said something about identity?

"What is a human being, a mammal? People are weird. We have made ourselves lord over it all and we can't manage it. I feel ashamed to be a human being."

How about stability?

"The sofa has its place where it belongs like in my parents' home or you have to drink half a litre of milk a day. I need rules, frames. I space out without frames. It shoots me out this way (*hand gesture*) or that (*hand gesture*). Everything is relative. Everything turns around, nothing is as it is and I really want that feeling!"

How does that feel?

"My body is buzzing, as if I am seeing with my entire body, spinning around. I can't think clearly, like in a trance-like state. It is calm, pleasant but impossible to act. I can't take care of a baby in that state!"

More about stability?

"It's because I have used myself as a crash test dummy. What happens if I do this or that to figure out things? What gives a meaning to my life? Find out what is really important about food and my body. I become angry, I have to figure it out! How do I know if P. is getting enough calcium? Do I need to become a nutritionist? I keep hitting a wall."

How does that feel?

"Busy, very busy, I don't feel prepared, there are chemicals in everything. Now I feel the blood drain from my head. I can't think anymore. Spinning, dragging me down. I can't move, I am paralysed. Deep grief actually, bottled up anger, incapacity, and powerlessness. There is a sadness in my chest (*weeps silently*), aloneness. A pressure in my chest, I can't breathe, I become superfluous, worthless. No stability, no fixed points, nothing is really there, I need a frame to be human within."

What happens without the frame?

"Everything is relative, just a lump of molecules without significance. I zoom out and see it all from high above. Why can't I figure it out down here? Stupid, silly. You have been given so many good tools but you don't use them."

What do you mean zoom out?

"Like using Google Earth (*gesture: like straight line from torso to high above head*) outside the planet. I feel dizzy. I would love to give P. a feeling of happiness of being human, that is why we created him."

How is it out there?

"Peaceful, calm, weightless, no problems. While I zoom out I hear a lot of voices. It's pure existence. It's me but not as a creature, no physical form. I recognise it all as one. I am just my thoughts, my eyes, no heart and no emotions, will but no warmth. Weightless, spinning, earth become a jigsaw puzzle, the pieces have to be moved around again for things to be ok. I feel no empathy, no emotions for the world. I have no body, I am just a head. It drives me nuts all this up and down, in and out of my body. I wish there was a ceiling for me (*hand gesture to indicate ceiling just above head*) My blood goes down (*gestures down*) and my energy goes up (*gestures up*) Two opposite energies, my head is weightless, my body is heavy. I wish I had a frame so I did not have to go up there and see it all from such as huge perspective."

You said you question everything?

"I think who cares? But that is not the right answer. It seems easier to just stay away, not participate, not to accept the task of being a human being. But that is our purpose, our task. I did not ask to be born."

How is it in space, out there?

"I am in one place, but at the same time everywhere. I am zooming back and forth, fast from place to place, with the speed of lightening."

What else?

"My milk is not flowing. I only have half of what he needs. The pregnancy was good, nature took over. Milk gives me digestive problems. I feel hot easily. I wake at 2 am. Sweating and cold, I feel warm but am cold to touch. I love salty liquorice (typically Danish thing). I love baked salmon and I dislike fatty food and pork. I am impatient, hot tempered, but people don't see it. People think I am 5–6 years older than I am."

Analysis

This patient's problem is that her field of focus is too big, she is not grounded. She feels she is outside mundane reality, seeing the whole planet, seeing the big picture all the time. This makes her feel a lack of stability and structure. She feels her head is drifting upwards, that there is no ceiling to stop her. She is confused about what she should do with her life on earth, with her newborn baby. She feels isolated, spinning, fat and ugly.

Rx: Helium 200C, single dose

Follow-up in August 2009

"The feeling of being a mother is now totally different. My son is wonderful, I really enjoy it and am much less worried. My focus is on being with him, playing and laughing. Now I have a totally different gut feeling, a grounded feeling. I see things from an everyday perspective and feel gravity now. I don't get lost in abstract thought, I stay here. I feel safer and have managed to establish routines. I have an important role in my son's life. It's important to me to be human, to be me. I am in my body now, not just in my head. My relationship to my mum is much better. I don't zoom out, away from earth. I don't end up out there as I used to. There is now a ceiling over my head. Breast feeding has been unproblematic. I still dream of atomic wars and still have a feeling of being fat. I still feel confused about my purpose in life, but I am further on in my plans to study."

Rx: Helium 10M

Follow-up in September 2009

"I had a strong reaction after taking the remedy, a deep old feeling of sadness. I know this feeling but it was much stronger. The next day I vomited 3–4 times. Since then I have been feeling really good. Better and better. Focusing is easy, I now focus on what is important right now. I feel more and more like me again. Like being a mother has been integrated. I feel I am present here, in my belly, a good feeling of gravity. Stability is even better. No dreams of atomic wars. My body feels like mine, not fat, just mine. I am able to plan my education. I feel more playful and inquisitive. I am less doubtful about my life choices. I am in charge of me; I don't get absorbed in things and lose myself unless I choose to. I don't get caught in the spinning trance. I am in my body now, not out in the universe. When I look at my son, I think wow, we are humans! We could have been something else.

The ceiling is a bit more open now. I can have big thoughts, but stay in myself. Lots of energy. When I listen to deep and meaningful radio programs I get the feeling of really understanding with the heart too, a nice warm feeling now. I feel love for humankind now, before I saw it all from the outside and thought, 'You are all fools'."

Comment

She did not need to repeat the remedy after that. A year and a half later she was still doing well.

CASE 8.7 'Spiritual wine'

Case from Shelly Been, Israel

The first consultation was in late November 2011. The patient was a man born in 1970 who is in a wheelchair due to limb-girdle muscular dystrophy.

He studies the Torah (Biblical studies – JS). He is overweight and wears a black skullcap. He used to have a vineyard and wants to publish a book on the subject. He taught music, guitar and became more religious at the age of 18. He closed the vineyard after several years, because there was a gap between his love of the profession and its application. From being 100% romance it became a business, which required a huge amount of investment and resources for the long run.

He studied spiritual studies for 5 years. He had a car accident. He didn't see a van when it crossed the road but this accident did not affect his health. The business didn't work before the grape harvest so he closed the business. The name of his vineyard was Har Nevo.[i]

"Making wine is fascinating. I caught the wine-making bug. It has something very internal about it, wine means secret in Gematria.[ii] My main complaint is a gap in application. A daily difficulty to

---

[i] Mount Nevo was the mountain that Moses climbed up from which to see Israel before dying. (JS)
[ii] According to Cabbalistic numerology. (JS)

function with the body as opposed to the internal will to achieve and manifest.

Everything I eat gets stuck (overweight). I desire meat and fish, farinaceous and fried food aggravate. One time I ate a falafel and felt I was floating outside of my body. My energy level is 5–6. My happiness level is 9. My confidence is usually strong, although there are times where it is not strong, as in relationships with women. I don't achieve full closeness, this is what I need to process. My self-love is 10. My self-acceptance is relative 10. Note: Patient uses standard terms from spiritual teacher, rather than his own words.

I sleep well and take no medication despite having a muscular dystrophy disease. I'm in a wheelchair because of the muscular dystrophy.

I want to develop a greater physical sensitivity. When I studied naturopathy I used to feel things. I felt the meridians before they were specified. Coffee aggravates my situation but I have difficulty in stopping it. I have a difficulty exposing myself.

When I was 24 I was very angry and took it out on my parents and friends. I was too good, they took it out on me and I was very cross."

Observation: looks up all the time.

"I used to be afraid of the dark and have unexplainable fears. Cockroaches are the only animal that causes a crazy reaction of fright."

Observation: restless fingers,

"I am stubborn and strict: My brother did something I didn't like and I didn't forgive him."

Observation: He seems totally unconnected to himself, nothing seems to move. Very hard and heavy. He speaks slowly and heavily.

"I was affected by a story of reincarnation where the conclusion was that if someone bothered a person during a previous life, he will continue to bother him in this reincarnation. I used to study in a yeshiva (religious school) and it was good. The muscular dystrophy put a stop to it. The disease put me into a very narrow radius and limited me. The limitations raised anger. The muscular dystrophy forces you to focus on certain things that you are required to handle. Questions like what did I do to deserve this?

Dreams: I saw myself standing and in my body I saw two very weak lights, which told me the reason for the muscular dystrophy. The lights were yellow-pink. I saw a certain rabbi who passed his hand over his beard and light went from the right brain to the left side of the body. The light went through him and expanded into my body. I understood it was The Ari (a famous Cabbalist) and that the dream was a *tikun* (*Note*: A message to help with rectification). I dreamt I saw a figure, an amazing man, with a face like a prophet and was told it was Abraham. Isaac was there also. Someone organised wood for a fire and the upper part of his body developed into a huge light. I was very frightened, a spiritual terror rather than a physical one, and I shouted for Yemima (spiritual guide). I also dreamt of Walt Disney cartoons. Another dream was of a candle lighting for departed souls.

As a boy I was very friendly. There was a sadness related to my body. I began walking at the very early age of 6 months. I walked in a strange manner and then the diagnosis of muscular dystrophy was made.

I am sensitive to my space being respected and I respect the space of others. I was very angry, it embarrassed me. Stuck in my brain. Loud house, made it hard to study.

At the age of 20 my body landed (*may be translated as took a dive, came down*), now my body is very weak. I returned from the yeshiva in Jerusalem in order to face my body and the social limitations. I had suicidal thoughts. I was limited with a wheelchair without an engine. I told God to take me, why are you keeping me here? I was not angry, I just wanted him to take me.

I like to do things in a perfect and total manner.

I get so hot that sometimes my body shivers and I feel stinging from the heat. During a half-sleep situation, I felt that my body suddenly increased in size and became heavy. I was out of my body and the body was left alone.

I have a desire for farinaceous food and wine. I like the wisdom in the wine. I'm interested in Jewish spirituality and Jewish identity. I have a fear of high places.

I used to have dandruff. I have had head pain in the past when I was angry. I wear glasses. I had Pneumonia twice. Sitting for long periods in the wheelchair causes sensitivity in the joints of my legs."

Rx Helium 6C daily

Follow-up in January 2011 (*after 40 days on Helium 6C*)
More energy in the body. He has completely stopped drinking coffee. He is less occupied by food and has a smaller appetite and capacity

for food. Eats healthier food, He has stopped eating fried and farin-aceous food and his digestion has improved. He feels like the cells in his brain are breathing. Smiles and laughs more. Financial issues are improving. The gap between application and the internal desire of the body is smaller. His energy has increased from 5–6 to 6.5 (out of 10). He feels better about women. He sleeps well and has lost a small amount of weight. His physical awareness is increased and he is less angry, more connected to his feelings. The pain in the joints of his legs has decreased. The pain in the shoulder has gone.

Follow-up in July 2011 (after not taking the remedy for 7 months)
He did not come back for a while but was feeling well. Feels much lighter in spirit and mentality. Manages to apply himself much more. All in all is happy. He has opened a spiritual study group with friends and studies most of the time. He feels more connected to his body with a better flow of energy. He is less occupied by food, eats less frequently and smaller amounts and is less inclined to temptations. Doesn't want to eat farinaceous and fried food. Eats less sweet food and margarine. The issue regarding the gap between the application and the desire has resolved itself. Digestion is good. Energy levels are up to 8 after starting 5–6. Regarding women, he feels that it is closer and more feasible. He accepts himself the way he is. In the past there was an illusion, the desire for perfection. He sleeps better and needs less sleep. Doesn't think about his physical awareness, the subject is no longer an issue. He is connected to his feelings and less angry. The pains in his body, have gone. He has understood that the pain in his legs was due to the fact that he did not stand on his feet for years and therefore the foot is naturally more sensitive. He feels the remedy is good for him since it makes him notice his body in a certain manner, pay more attention to the physical system. It has something more intentional and real.

Rx: Helium 6C daily for 5 weeks

Follow up in September 2011
Everything feels better. Lost 5.5kgs. The systems in the body are more connected, feeling more alert. Underwent a spiritual experience and understands why he has been eating so much.

Is eating less. Sensations from his childhood have returned, where as a child he did not want to eat and his parents forced him. Is less hungry and does not feel the desire to eat fried food. The digestion has improved.

Observation: seems much lighter, laughs more.

Financially he sees that he needs much less and has the possibility of doing good for others with his money, which gives him more abundance.

Feels things are much more flowing, can apply much more, like a dam has opened.

Has not got a relationship yet, however knows more what he wants.

The sleep is more concentrated, does not need to sleep so much.

Is less angry, the block of anger has disseminated to many things, each case is treated individually and therefore it is handled in a totally different manner.

There are no pains in his muscles.

Rx: Helium 6C daily, diluted in water

In November 2011 the patient reported continued improvement.

Case 8.8 'In between to be or not to be'

Case from Katrin Sigwart, Germany[i] (edited for brevity)
In the summer of 2005 a female patient came to see me.

"When I called to make an appointment for the case-taking I was in much worse shape than I have been for a long time. It's like becoming totally destructive. I badmouth myself. I question everything I do: my motherhood, my relationship with my partner, my behaviour in the relationship, but also my partner, my job, if I'm doing well in my job, or well enough. Everything becomes meaningless.

What touches me very much at other times as well is the fate of other human beings: human beings starving, people that are being tortured or persecuted or abused. This hits me as if I had experienced it with my own body. Tears come to my eyes; it really hurts me. That's

---

[i] Also appearing in Schlingesiepen-Brysch, I. *The Source in Homeopathy. Cosmic Diversity and Individual Talent – Source-based Homeopathy Volume I*. Kandern: Narayana Verlag; 2009.

something that is almost always present, this compassion for others, and it becomes almost unbearable. Then I think I don't want to live anymore, I don't want to deal with all this anymore. It's horrible, it gets so extreme. I've sat at home for hours and wept over the state this world is in. We have a housekeeper and I really have a problem with her, with the fact that she has less than I do and I always want to give her something, share with her, give away some of what I have. If I buy cheese, for example, then I give her a piece. It's often hard for me to charge money in my practice. I very often give sessions to people for free when I know that they don't have much.

What I'm disturbed by, especially physically, is my tiredness. It's not as bad as it used to be, like total exhaustion, but I'm tired a lot. What has caused a lot of worries for me recently is that I have lost my dedication, my zest for life and for many things. A zest for life doesn't exist anymore.

I used to care a lot about everybody associated with me being well. I always had the wellbeing of not only my family but everybody who was with me in mind. I felt responsible and guilty for their state. I think this comes from the situation that my mother wasn't at all well when she was carrying me. Two of my brothers before me died shortly after birth. Then I came. I feel like you realise that in the uterus. That's why I've always tried to please everybody.

I can remember that once as a child I was really irate, so that they put me under a cold shower to calm me down. I can remember such fits of anger and the trigger was always that I felt treated unfairly.

I was sent to a boarding school at the age of ten. I was completely lost, extremely homesick, felt totally lost and left behind and became anorexic after a while."

What do you wish to change the most out of all you've mentioned?

"These destructive phases where I don't know my way around at all and this being restrained."

Describe restrained.

"Before the anorexia began at about 14 or 15, I began to flirt, to experiment with young men. I would have liked to go out with different men and to smooch with them. I can remember my brother commenting negatively on that. I was so shocked by that, that I restrained myself immediately. I didn't live to the full in the way I would have liked to, just trying out how it is. I think I had a distinct sensuality and sexuality that I already began to choke back at that time. I denied my sexuality for years and didn't experience it or only in a very limited way. So I restrained myself very much.

I know that I was quite brash. I realised that I hurt people and began to control that. You could say that the anorexia was to make myself less, make myself smaller, reduce my needs. It must have come from a feeling that I'm not good the way I am, I'm not right the way I am. Of course that affected my body. If there were parties or we went on a trip with the school, I always had the feeling that the others were excluding me. But they also gave me the feeling I was giving myself airs, showing off.

I've always had the feeling that I'm not attractive, I'm ugly, nobody wants me. The other girls were always more interesting and that also hurt me very much, that too was reflected by my anorexia. In my practice I only ever see what I've done badly. I never see the successes. Somebody else has to point them out to me. I don't have the self-confidence. In my practice I'm calm and have patience and am focused on what I'm doing. But with my other interests I have such a tattered feeling, wanting to be everywhere."

Describe tattered and being everywhere.

"Being able to do everything. To suck in life, live life to the full, like without sleeping."

Describe to suck in life. Imagine I don't know the word.

"Sensual pleasures is the first thing that comes to my mind, that is sucking in, kissing, eating, drinking, being present through all your pores. Like a huge mouth, a huge opening, that can taste, take up, drink, sense everything. Or huge eyes, huge pores. Like enclosing the world, enclosing the world with your whole body."

Describe enclosing the world with your whole body.

"That is fusing actually. Fusing is to become one. To sense every-thing that is there, to be in interaction with it. It is a constant reaction to what is all around me. Again, like a flowing movement. To become one."

Describe becoming one, fusing.

"Not being separated, now it's gone, this feeling of fusing."

Describe the opposite of fusing.

"Alone or separated. I'm sensing something very unpleasant, itching, now. I sense my body like my separated body. It has very sharp contours, just as if I'm being marked out by a pair of compasses, contoured. And the other thing is not feeling any of that any more, but fusing like this. No contours exist. Instead, it just flows. I can't describe it. It is not only to fuse with the earth but with the entirety of space. It is not existence anymore, it is as if there was no consciousness. As if consciousness were separation."

Consciousness were separation?

"Somehow I've got the feeling that thinking is an incredible obstacle, an impediment to being, to simply being."

Describe being, simply being.

"I can't picture that. Like a white mass but it is not mass. It isn't heavy, it's very light, but I can't say it's like air. It can also be black."

What is being?

"It is air, a mass that isn't heavy. It's got something to do with this not wanting to exist anymore. It's simply everything that exists as a being, as a person, as an animal, as a human, as a plant. Everything is simply linked to this pain or to this suffering. And there has to be a state where this does not exist."

Describe this state.

"This me and you and everything else that takes place in the world."

What exactly does not exist there?

"I'm afraid of dying because I'm afraid of once again being somewhere where I don't know my way around, where I don't know the rules. Where I'm alone, where I have to go through the arduous process of finding my way, where there is again this being separated."

Describe being separated, the phenomenon itself without it referring to you.

"That something consists of separate parts instead of being a whole. Now I've just seen a sphere that other spheres circulate around, and then I came to think of the black hole, which scares me incredibly."

Describe the black hole.

"The black hole where there is simply nothing anymore, horrifying."

What is horrifying?

"That nothingness."

Describe nothingness. What is this nothingness?

"I can't think that."

What is so horrifying?

"That I can't think that."

What can't you think?

"Nothing, I cannot think that. There exists something else between our existence and the nothingness; there is an intermediary state that is without this individual consciousness. It is connected, where everything flows and merges together."

Describe this intermediary state between our existence and the nothingness.

"That is a feeling of being united without being an individual, without demands, without ego."

Describe being united, the phenomenon itself, being united without being an individual.

"That is a state of, I can't say of not experiencing, but not of experiencing either. Simply being without particular demands."

Describe being without particular demands.

"I constantly have an image that I can't describe, because it is not a picture but a feeling, but also not really a feeling. It is a state, a white mass that isn't really any mass either, because it isn't heavy and still has a certain substance."

What kind of mass could that be, white, not heavy, no real mass?

"Maybe some kind of gas but one that does not evaporate, that is held together somehow. I'm always thinking of helium although I have no idea at all what helium is."

So what is helium?

"It is something relatively heavy that still floats, that won't evaporate, but is held together. But it isn't solid, it has no substance in that sense. Something that holds together but has no body, no form; that fills in everything one can think of.

A stone comes to my mind, a mountain, an empty volcano, a wire. I experienced states when I became incredibly ill, I became unconscious and then woke up and thought I would dissolve, and that was always linked to incredible fear. I vomited terribly. Then I used to lie for three days without moving, without eating or drinking. Afterwards I was well again. I feel the brakes are being put on life, to leave out what is total about it, let go. Simply being as it is, uncontrolled.

It isn't water, but something more intensive, thicker. It still has a strong dynamism but is nevertheless soft. It is not completely uncontrolled. It doesn't drown in the mass I'm talking about here. It has its own form, but that form is flowing. I have a feeling the remedy is something like an element. I thought it could be Helium. That wasn't by deduction, it just came to me because I had this picture, like in the universe."

Fusing, becoming one. To sense everything that there is, to be in interaction. It is a feeling of being united without being an individual, without demands, without ego: a state of simply being and a state of nothingness. She then describes an intermediary state between being and not being. The theme of being or not being is the leitmotif in the first period (row) of the periodic table which holds Hydrogen and Helium. Hydrogen has the theme of not yet existing. Helium describes the actual conception, the moment between non-existence and the beginning of existence.

Rx. Helium 50M

The patient was given a 50M because as she emphasised in many communications after the initial case-taking, one of her main problems was the disturbance of her life energy. A 50M has a healing effect on the life energy itself.

Follow-up in July 2005

"Slowly but steadily a deep inner calmness and satisfaction spread within me. It was like floating and smiling and the feeling was everything is good. Less thinking in the sense of pondering, greater reassurance in my activities in my practice, a greater distance and delimitation towards friends. The tiredness has got very slowly less but my exhaustion has been gone for a year now."

Rx: Helium 50M

Continuation of case

The next time she took another dose of the 50M, she sounded more sober.

"This time it took longer for the pleasant change to set in again and it wasn't as noticeable. What has remained is the ability to set boundaries between myself and others without fear of isolation. I have also noticed from the first time I took it up to now an increasing ability to express myself openly without thinking a lot about it and without being afraid of inconveniencing somebody else through this, or of being to blame for somebody else's indisposition. In the past this had always been a great problem for me."

In February 2006 the patient took another 50M dose during a minor relapse of her state, which had been good until that time, apparently too early. Over a period of weeks her old mental state returned (like before the treatment).

"I realised that because I was in a bad state over many weeks: for the first time I was just as I had been before the case-taking, except for my despair about the suffering of the world. That did not reappear in the old intensity."

I recognise the patient's observation from other patients who have taken an exactly fitting remedy either too early or in an overdose: old mental troubles return as an overreaction and die away again when the effects of the overdose peter out.

The remedy's effect ran out again in the spring of 2007 and after taking it once more, she reports on the months March to August 2007 as follows:

"It was as if in a flow. It was without any destination. The road was beautiful: simply a rejoicing in life. The case-taking was so deep (in the cases I undertook in my practice). It was such a feeling of love for human beings. I wasn't afraid of death that is otherwise such a terrible subject for me. If I died, I would not be separated from the children and the others. This world and the beyond are one."

In October and November 2007 the effects of her remedy ran out again, which she realised this from the worsening of her state of mind again. Her old fears and her feeling of non-existence returned for a few nights. Because her life energy remained balanced, she took a 10M for the first time. Since then until today (March 2008), in her own words she has been, "Very well again, give or take some minor ups and downs that come with everyday life."

CASE 8.9 'Abused'

Case from Jeremy Sherr
This case has only been treated for three months. I decided to include it because there is much to learn about Helium from it, even though it has gone to other remedies and may well need others still. Helium bought about a profound improvement and a first step in of the healing journey, after many other remedies failed to help. This case

is far from finished, and there are many issues that will still have to be dealt with due to the difficult history.

Young Man, has had many homeopathic remedies throughout his life with no help.

"As a child I experienced serious sexual abuse for a sustained period of time. The legacy of this limits my life. Here is one moment of the past, though unfortunately there were many others. . . .

I am taped up, this is a game. Then a deal is done that if I can get out, I don't have to do anything, but if I can't I do. I believe this is fair and I can, so they say, 'see if you can get out'. So I struggle and struggle and then I'm exhausted. I'm broken so then I have to perform a sexual act. Then they leave me in the room, stuck and alone. All abuse has a bondage theme.

I am haunted by the memories of the past, and when the memories are most prevalent, I will have adult sexual fantasies with a bondage theme which I hate.

In life, I feel I am always stuck, waiting, locked, not moving forwards, never quite breaking through. I always feel like I'm looking out of a window at a moving world, when I'm not. I spend my life not wanting to be where I am and fearing the passing of time, wanting more, and not getting it. Wanting to be bigger, stronger, richer, some-where else.

In my body, I can't lose weight, I feel small and exhausted and because of this and the grip of the past, I don't do intimacy.

In a nutshell, I can't lose weight, I can't be intimate, I can't realise my potential, I hate not having enough money, and I don't want to be where I am.

I feel I could be infinitely possible if I could only wash away the trappings of the past.

It is so hard, so painful. I am looking for a breakthrough and move-ment.

Horrendous period of childhood sustained abuse. Memories haunt-ing me. Devastated by the past. When the memory comes back I gets sexual fantasies that I hate. Devastated by them, like I am fighting myself.

I am fat, and friendly. I work very hard but never realise anything. Always the one who just misses, trapped in so many ways, I move away from realising anything, I feel isolated. I want with my whole heart and soul to move, but find myself stuck. Stuck with relationships, always looking through a window into the world. I work so hard and isolate myself. I feel terrible about me body. I feel physically stunted, small hands and feet, genitalia, short, overweight."

Observation: He is a charming, open and self aware person, seems very capable.

"So sad, I want to move forward. I have no thunder. I try so hard and push and push and always thrown back, cant actualise anything, no destination, no moment of realisation. I feel the passing of time, getting older, people getting older. I can't bear the days passing without something moving. Everything is a struggle. I come so close, so much potential to live and to succeed, but I don't, I don't live in the moment, live in a dream of future but regret of past.

I hate inactivity.

I struggle, been very low. I grieve about things, shout into a pillow Muscles cracking.

Bubbling in abdomen, bladder.

I feel hemmed in, tight, closed off, locked, shrouded. Looking out through glass, can't speak. I work, I am sociable, involved, but there is an isolation.

Sustained sexual abuse, bondage, didn't tell anybody, I didn't know what was normal

I believed it was my thought or freewill or doing to please. Since adolescence I have fought thinking about it, about where my sexuality has been broken. Constant struggle, step back from any opportunity of intimacy. I feel inadequate in inacy, a freak and full of distrust, unwillingness to take part, feels tainted.

Looking for a normal relationship until the dark thoughts hit, don't want to engage, inner battle, I fight it, partly not engaging which is tragic.

It was not my parents, they were very good, I adore my parents, they were not involved, redeeming. My abusers could be comforting, but evil.

I never felt anger, very hard, don't get angry. They convinced me a lot of it was games, from age 3, games, seeing if I can get out but I could not.

I yearn for something more, like a hunger, I put a lot on money, associate it with safety, maybe a position of power to be needed. I get bored quickly if things aren't happening.

I try to be the best at everything, come close, yearning for something bigger then I am. I like to do things well, creating but can't manifest

I work for months on a project but can't find the peace or joy. At the moment when it looks possible and I get terrified – the intersection between possibility and reality. I can't reach beyond that, a point I can't get at. I can't reach anger. If I can get there I would be hit, something bad would happen

Lose hair when stressed.

Tension jaw.

Eat too much, crave food.

Spots on skin, skin feels thin.

Dislocate joints easily, knees ankles wrists.

Palms sweat.

A lot of dreams: being at gun point, guns. Also good dreams – flying or weightless dancing, effortless hand stands, I am light, can do hand stands and roll over, lightness. Flying high and weightless.

Dream of them and their house to prove to people it has happened, prove or disprove to myself. Dream penises, sexually inappropriate dreams, try to call the police try to dial but cannot.

Dream castles like buildings around water, dream the incoming tide.

I tell myself a lot of stories, wizards and dragons scenarios, I live in my head when bored and frightened. A hero or safe, envisage things. Magical themes, strong, extra abilities, command fire, be strong, sword fights, mythical wars.

Feel like I want to run around, want movement, I want something to change, I want the glass to shatter, to go through, like a knife through butter and movement. Always looking out of a window, then and now, locked stuck and trapped, not actualising anything.

Fear passing of time, fear people dying. Time passing, life moving on and I'm stuck.

Mother has a long labour with me, rushed to hospital, fearful, traumatic.

At times I almost leave my body, through my vertex.

I am very academic but also dyslexic."

Rx: Helium 1m

Follow up one month later

"Brilliant!! Amazing, sexual fantasies gone, much better! I feel much stronger!

I am pushing forward really hard. I sleep better, manage better – brilliant.

The remedy has really lifted me. I am feeling much more level, normal, and able to push forward. The sexual fantasies have not haunted me this month, which is revolutionary. And I've been sleeping less haunted nights too.

Eating much much better, much less from 100 meals a day to 2 meals, always struggled with that. I exercise more, doing things differently, feel easy, things showing glimmer of possibility.

I managed things much better, fantastic!!

The remedy has done great things, but this fear has come up.

I am knocking on the door, see the fear differently.

After the remedy many dreams of coming downstairs, then fighting people and afraid.

I have gone further than I could ever imagine with this remedy, and now it has bought me to a point of great fear.

At the moment, when things happen or are about to happen, the reaction to this is fear. So I must STOP, shut down – this is not a conscious action, but unconsciously I want to stop until whatever's happening does stop. It feels like it could turn to hell and then it actually does. The fear feels like being struck. I feel frozen like I will just stay still, not seeing, feeling sick, like I want to flinch, mentally consumed by it all.

Dreams: I'm on the top of a hill and I'm walking down with water flowing beside me. Suddenly I'm back at the top of the hill. This happens three times, with the water flowing stronger each time. Then as I'm walking down, there is a black hole where all the water is flowing. I try not to get sucked into the hole. But I must shelter in the entrance, or I will get struck by lightning from the storm outside. So I'm trying not to get sucked down, or struck.

There is still a block- but different, when something happens I feel exposed, vulnerable out of control, very scared.

Fantastic remedy, and now a change of emphasis, more fear."

Rx Aconite 200c

Note: After some deliberation I decided to change the remedy to what was appropriate for the moment. My understanding, based on the story and dreams, was that he had begun to incarnate but as he approached birth the fear of danger came up strongly, reminiscent of his mother's traumatic experience during his birth. This is echoed in the dream of falling through the hole with the possibility of being struck by lightning. In this change of remedy I am following Hahnemann's instructions on the second prescription (§162–§184). The case may point to a complimentary relationship between Helium and Aconite.

Email after two weeks
All fear gone.

Rx: Helium 1M

Follow up six weeks later
"The fear is much better, gone. It went after Aconite.

Helium opened everything up, transformed me, taken away all the darkness and negativity. The horrible sexual fantasies have gone. I have much more energy, exercising, closer to people. Life is moving."

9

HELIUM MM ANALOGY, BIOLOGY, COSMOLOGY

This chapter is my personal arrangement and interpretation of the proving symptoms, especially the more obscure ones. Many of these come from Silvie, and I am once again grateful for her amazing capacity to hear the gentle whispers of a proving and translate them into poetry. She is the channel for most of this information, while I am merely an interpreter. I opted to place this section after the cases, because most cases can be solved using knowledge obtained from the earlier sections of this book. The sections that follow are intended for the esoterically adventurous. If you decide to ignore this section you will still have an almost full use of the remedy. In fact I almost recommend that you don't read it. I just needed to write it. If this is not your game please proceed to chapter 11: *Dimensions*.

The higher we climb the wider we see. Being the MM level of perception, this investigation relates to the collective realm as well as to Helium as an individual remedy.

Note that this chapter contains only selected quotes from the proving. Please refer to the Appendix 'MM proving symptoms' for other related symptoms, and to the full proving for the unedited chronological sequence.

In writing this chapter I was often reminded of the cabbalistic story in which four sages entered a 'Pardes' or orchard, a Hebrew acronym representing a mystical journey through the different levels of personal awareness and cosmic experience.[i] There are four levels to this journey: the simple explanation, hints pertaining to a hidden meaning, the deeper search or inquiry, and the highest level, that of the mystic secret. One of the four sages died, one went insane, one became a heretic and only the fourth made it back safely.

---

[i] *The Talmud* (Chagiga 14b), *Zohar* (I, 26b) and *Tikunei Zohar* (Tikun 40) report the following incident regarding four Mishnaic Sages.

Or in the words of Albert Einstein:[1]

A thought that sometimes makes me hazy:
Am I – or are the others crazy?

In this chapter I elaborate on the most complex aspects of the proving. It was only after extensive study and by arranging and rearranging the themes that I was able to unravel some of the secrets hidden within. I have left some of the more complicated aspects for an MMM chapter, which will appear in the ultimate book of this series. What I have written below is my analysis and synthesis of the proving facts. I do not profess to understand it all, far from it, nor do I think this is necessary or possible. There are still many secrets. As Silvie says in the proving:

A fine thread of light. Do not unravel the mysteries. Wisdom and understanding, yet do not delve. Have faith, do not expose our origins.

This journey involves an exploration of the analogies between the proving of Helium, physics, biology and esoteric knowledge. **I am only offering a brief exposition of these vast bodies of knowledge as they are far too extensive to cover in depth; moreover the information is available elsewhere. My intention is to use the Helium proving to enhance the synthesis of these subjects. It is up to each reader to further study each subject should he or she wish to do so.**

My purpose is twofold: First, to draw your attention to certain parallels within and between these topics. Second, to develop new ideas based on the unique Helium information which was previously unavailable.

I will be comparing four different factors: the proving of Helium, the account of creation according to modern physics, the biology of reproduction and esoteric cosmology. Esoteric cosmology will be represented by Mishna and Cabbala, Jewish Biblical interpretations and mysticism. I use this esoteric approach both because it seemed to offer the most fitting metaphors to the Helium proving and because it is closest to my roots. I do retain the liberty of new approaches to traditional cabbasitic concepts, otherwise I would just be reiterating what is already known. This liberty is is an integral part of cabbalistic tradition.

I have no doubt that there are many other related bodies of knowledge, both scientific and esoteric, coming from many traditions, that would be worth studying in this context but they are beyond the scope of this book.

You may wonder what these comparisons have to do with the proving of Helium. I hope this will become clear as we continue. I will begin with an introduction to creation as it is perceived by modern physics. To understand Helium one must understand Hydrogen, and to understand both Hydrogen and Helium, one must understand the process by which they were created, the origins of the universe.

So let us begin at the beginning.

Physics: From the Big Bang to stars

According to modern physics, the universe began with the Big Bang, an explosion of an extremely dense and contracted substance called a singularity. This is said to have occurred some 13.7 billion years ago, give or take a day.

With appropriate instrumentation, one can still observe the remnants of the primeval light that emanated from that explosion, which dates back to the origins of time. The approximate sequence of events after the Big Bang is as follows:

- During the first 10^{-43} seconds, the **four** fundamental forces of physics are unified (gravity, weak, strong and electromagnetic). Temperature: 10^{32} Kelvin. At 10^{-43} seconds, gravity splits from the other forces.
- In the first 10^{-35} seconds, quarks and anti-quarks dominate the universe. Temperature drops to 10^{27} Kelvin. The strong force separates from the weak and electromagnetic forces. At 10^{-12} seconds the four forces become distinct.
- At 0.01 seconds, electrons and positrons form as the temperature drops to 10^{11} Kelvin. After 1 second, the universe becomes transparent to neutrinos (sub-atomic particles with zero charge and zero mass produced in nuclear fusion reactions), which from this point on hardly interact with matter.
- Three minutes after the Big Bang, the temperature dropped to 10^{9}K. Protons and neutrons combine to form what will become the nuclei of elements (mostly hydrogen and helium).
- 300,000 years later the temperature has dropped to 3000K and the electrons are captured by nuclei to form atoms. The universe becomes transparent to light (photons stop interacting with free electrons) resulting in the formation of cosmic background radiation.
- After 1 billion years, the temperature is 20K. Galaxies and stars have begun to form via gravitational contraction of the universe. After a few billion years our galaxy forms, and about 10 billion years after the Big Bang, the sun and earth form. After 13 billion years we finally reach the present background temperature of about 3K.

Cabbala

> Science without religion is lame, religion without science is blind.
>
> Albert Einstein[2]

Much of Cabbala deals with the creation of the world and the souls that inhabit it, hence it frequently relates to the provings of Hydrogen and Helium, the first elements of our universe, whose provings depict the creation and evolution of the soul. There are many Cabalistic accounts of creation. I will be referring mostly to the Zohar, the main tome of Cabbala, and to the version developed by Rabbi Isaac Luria, known as the Ari (1534–1572).[3]

According to Cabbala, in the beginning the universe did not exist, there was only the infinite light of God. The creator was alone, occupying all space with limitless and infinite light. The existence of any entity in addition to this light would have been impossible, because this would have constituted a limitation of God's infinity. He could not bestow his influence because there was no one to receive it. To enable the universe to exist required an act of 'contraction', a withdrawal on the part of God. God retracted the light in all directions from a certain singular place (a dot) leaving a circular void.

The opening line of the *Zohar* (Genesis) begins:

> In the beginning of the King's authority, the Lamp of Darkness engraved a hollow in the Supernal Luminescence. Know that before the emanated things were emanated and the created things were created, the pure divine light filled all existence. . . . The Eyn Sof contracted himself into a central point with His light in the middle. He contracted this light and then removed Himself to the sides encircling the point at the center. . . . This contraction, equidistant all around the point in the center, formed a void in such a way that the vacuum was spherical in all sides in equal measure. . . . Then, one straight line **descended** from the light of Eyn Sof.[4]

Essentially God's first creation was that of a lack, a void. This suggests that true creation occurs not by doing or intervening but by letting things go. God rules the world not by doing, but by 'not doing'.

The *Tao Te Ching* puts it like this:[5]

> Thirty spokes share the wheel's hub;
> It is the centre hole that makes it useful.
> Shape clay into a vessel;
> It is the space within that makes it useful.
> Cut doors and windows for a room;
> It is the holes which make it useful.
> Therefore profit comes from what is there;
> Usefulness from what is not there.

And

> The world is ruled by letting things take their course.
> It cannot be ruled by interfering.

The universe is now a void. In this regard it is interesting to study the proving of Vacuum by Nuala Eising.[6] There are several similarities to Helium, including mirror images, sense of purpose or lack of purpose.

The void has a 'desire to receive'; hence God could bestow his goodness into it. The word Cabbala literally means 'receiving'. Only a faint imprint of light remained in the void, creating a blueprint for all creation (cf. Kent's 'simple substance' described in Chapter 1 – *Introduction*).

In the centre of this void remained a single dot of light. This dot is the smallest possible point and cannot be divided or reduced. It is the centre and the essence of creation, the common denominator of all dots from which the universe is composed. Within this dot is folded the potential for the ten cabbalistic vessels, the precursors of the tree of life.

According to the thirteenth-century cabbalist, Moses de Leon (1250–1305), who is quoted by Daniel Matt in his book *God and the Big Bang:*[7]

> The beginning of existence is the secret concealed point. This is the beginning of all the hidden things, which spread out from there and emanate, according to their species. From a single point you can extend the dimensions of all things. Similarly, when the concealed arouses itself to exist, at first it brings into being something the size of the point of a needle; from there it generates everything

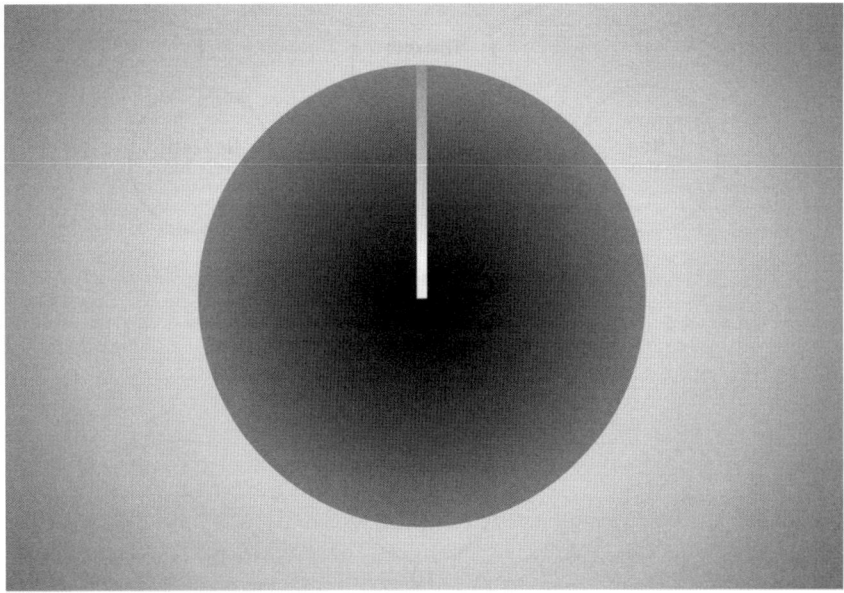

Figure 9.1 *The ray of light flowing through the void*

Into the centre of this void flows the ray of light (see Figure 9.1), retaining God's presence in the universe.

As the material world results primarily from the absence of God's light, it appears to be devoid of God's presence. However we are not totally forsaken. Into this void flows a ray of God's light. This ray, and the faint imprint of light which remains, signify the continual presence of God in creation. They bestow every being with the awareness that God is within us all, continuously creating anew. The linear ray of light represents the masculine, while the circular and delicate imprint of light in the void

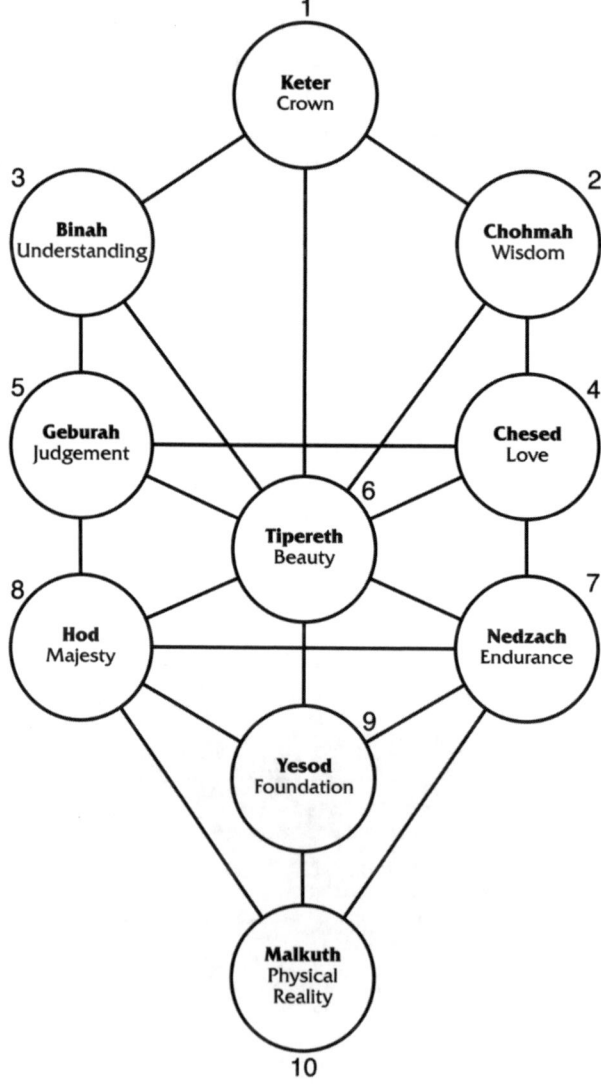

Figure 9.2 The tree of life

represents the feminine. It is the interaction of these two forces, line and circle, that unify to create the spiral motion which animates the world.

The ray of light shines through and fills the ten vessels (or *Sephirot*), representing the vehicles through which God interacts with the universe. These vessels are arranged in the form of the Tree of Life (depicted in Figure 9.2), illustrating the sequence and process by which the universe comes into being.

Initially, as the ray of God's light passes through the first three Sephirot, they are able to contain the intense energy. As the light surges through the remaining seven Sephirot, however, it becomes too powerful to be contained, and the vessels crack and shatter. This concept is known as 'the breaking of the vessels'. As a result of this shattering, the light is scattered into sparks. Initially there were 288 sparks, which later divided and sub-divided into many thousands.

The collective mission of humanity is to gather together these sparks to reform the original light. This can be achieved by good deeds and the fulfilling of holy commandments, a process known as *'tikkun olam'* (fixing, amending the world). Only by this process can the seven broken Sephirot regain their former perfection. Until the process is complete, the seven lower aspects of creation are shattered and the sparks of heavenly light remain scattered throughout the universe.

It is remarkable to find the following image in the Helium proving:

I woke suddenly like in a dream, and there were huge cracks appearing in the walls of the house. The vessel was shattering and it could be seen from the inside.

Physics, Cabbala and the provings of Hydrogen and Helium

One of the main premises of the Hermetic tradition, Cabbala and other philosophies is *'as above so below'*.[8]

In other words, all that exists in the physical world has a counterpart in the spiritual world. The cabbalist explanation of creation has remarkable similarities to that favoured by modern science. There are several parallels to be drawn between these bodies of knowledge to the provings of Hydrogen and the noble gases.

In the cabbalist story of creation, the universe begins with the limitless energy of God. Chinese philosophy calls this *Tao*. This primal state of being is not documented in modern physics. In physics, nothing is recorded or understood prior to the Big Bang; the singularity simply existed.

> A blinding spark flashed within the concealed of the concealed, from the mystery of the Infinite, a cluster of vapour in formlessness. . . . Under the impact of breaking through, one high and hidden point shone. Beyond that point nothing is known. So it is called Beginning[9]

One might say God's circular contraction is the Big Bang. The explosion of the condensed universe, which continues to expand until today, is analogous to the expanding void, the 'negative' of God's contraction. The faint imprint of God's light which remains in the void refers to background radiation. In the centre of this void is a singular dot in which all things are contained, corresponding to the singularity of physics.

A more detailed description of the parallels between Cabbalah and the big bang may be found in *The Secret Doctrines of the Kabbalah* by Leonara Leet.[10]

The Biblical account of creation begins with the following words

In the beginning, God created the heavens and the earth

In Hebrew this verse is written as follows:

בְּרֵאשִׁית, בָּרָא אֱלֹהִים, אֵת הַשָּׁמַיִם, וְאֵת הָאָרֶץ.

There are numerous interpretations of this verse, probably more than any other in the Bible. It is widely acknowledged in Cabbala that the first letter of the bible, the Bet (ב) is the source of creation. Bet is the preposition 'in' as 'in the beginning'. Other texts interpret it as 'by means of the beginning'. Note that the dot in the centre of the Bet is grammatically significant.

My interpretation is that the dot in the middle of the first letter *Bet* represents the singularity. The letter Bet literally means 'House', which is apparent in the way the letter is shaped. As such it signifies the containing principle. The *Bet* encircles the dot. Thus the first letter of the bible graphically depicts the creator withdrawing his light, leaving a singularity in the middle. Perhaps the letter Bet stands for Big Bang.

Sparks and photons

Let us now return to the Cabbala's shattering of the vessels. Initially the vessels are able to contain the light. However after the briefest period of time, the seven lower vessels shatter leaving only the three top vessels intact. Following the shattering of the vessels, God's light is fragmented into sparks. In order to restore the original light, these sparks have to be rectified and gathered together as one.

> I have seen that all those sparks flash from the High Spark, hidden of all hidden. All are levels of enlightenment. In the light of each and every level there is revealed what is revealed. All those lights are connected: this light to that light, that light to this light, one shining into the other, inseparable, one from the other.[11]

A fragment of a second after the Big Bang, the universe consisted of a 'cosmic soup' of photons, neutrons, electrons, protons and anti-particles. Photons are the basic unit of all electromagnetic phenomena, in other words they are particles of light. Like the sparks of Cabbala, we may say that photons are fragments of the universal soul.

Hydrogen

Photons produce particles, particles evolve into elements and elements fuse and react with each other. A few minutes after the Big Bang, photons and other particles began to form atomic nuclei, mostly hydrogen and helium. The initial ratio was about 75 percent hydrogen to 25 percent helium (i.e. 3:1), which is similar to the hydrogen to helium ratio today.

The homeopathic proving of Hydrogen describes the soul's initial separation from God. In the proving we can clearly perceive echoes of the Cabbalist account of creation (according to the Lurianic tradition). Initially the universe is filled with God's light and love, which contracts, thus separating God from his creation. A feint light remains, the 'collective sea of souls', and a ray of light penetrates and charges this void. This is followed by the shattering of the vessels and the scattering of sparks, leaving a fragmentation of souls that must be painstakingly healed. In homeopathic terms, this event marks the beginning of psora. In paragraph 103 of the *Organon*, Hahnemann describes this fragmentation as follows:[12,13]

> The psoric symptoms of each individual are] a dissevered, as it were, portion of the totality of the symptoms which constitute the entire extent of this malady.

The following symptoms are all taken from the Hydrogen proving:

I felt in the presence of a totally pure energy, like meeting God and feeling totally unworthy or like meeting a lover and feeling unworthy – realising all the mistakes of a lifetime. This pure energy was around for some time protecting me. I feel this unification cleared out lifetimes of symptomatology for me. The joining with this energy was as if a male energy joined with me sexually, but with no desire, pleasure or pain involved. This unification with the male energy lasted quite a few days – I'm not used to seeing myself as a man. The morning after this unifying with the higher presence, I collapsed in emotional overflow. All my grief and pain came out. I was doubled up on the floor and I went into a deep state of catharsis. It is not possible to describe where I went as there are no concepts applicable. I felt overflowing love for humanity and wanted to give everything away. My mind turned to the Buddha. It was like seeing the complete picture instead of fragmented bits.

I feel I have moved into a different state of consciousness and there aren't any guiding posts or means of navigation, a bit like being lost in space.

Feeling of visiting another dimension and having to come back here where it's all the same as it was before.

The photons, fragments of God's universal light, have created the particles that make up a hydrogen atom, symbolising a fragment of the universal soul. So we can say that photons are analogous to the sparks of light that combine to make up the soul.

The Hydrogen proving shows us that the primordial Hydrogen has a totally homogenous sexuality, which manifests as a gender identity crisis and confusion between left and right sides, both apparent in the proving. Thus Hydrogen represents an aspect of the collective soul, separated from God but as yet undifferentiated and non-individualised.

Nucleosynthesis

Hydrogen fuses into helium in a multi-stage process termed nucleosynthesis. In the basic hydrogen fusion cycle, four hydrogen nuclei (protons) come together to form a helium nucleus. This is the simple version of the story. In fact there are also electrons, neutrinos and photons involved in the fusion of hydrogen into helium. The by-product of this fusion is an enormous amount of light and heat, the power behind all stars including our sun.

It should be stated that there are two forms of Helium nucleosythesis, the proton-proton cycle which occurs in smaller stars and the CNO (carbon–nitrogen–oxygen) cycle which occurs in larger ones. As nucleosyntheis in our sun is based on the proton-proton cycle I will refer to that in our analogy. The process is illustrated in Figure 9.3.

The proton-proton chain begins with two protons (^1H) colliding to form a nucleus of deuterium (^2H). Any time such fusion takes place, a tiny amount of mass is turned into a comparatively huge amount of energy. When the two protons fuse to make the deuterium, one of the protons turns into a neutron and releases energy in the form of a positron (e^+) and a neutrino (v); the positron annihilates with an electron, creating two

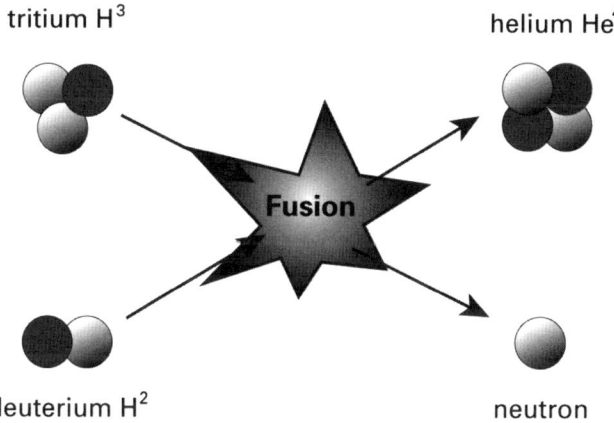

Figure 9.3 *Nucleosynthesis: The fusion of hydrogen into helium*

gamma rays (γ). The deuterium then combines with another proton, releasing a gamma ray and giving a nucleus of helium-3 (^{3}He). Finally, the helium-3 nucleus fuses with another helium-3 to form normal helium (^{4}He). This last step sets free two protons to start the whole process again. The gamma rays produced in the proton-proton reaction take 1 to 10 million years to work their way out from the star's core, being scattered numerous times and losing energy as they go, until they emerge from the surface as rays of light and heat. Inside the sun, about 655 million tons of hydrogen are converted into 650 million tons of helium every second.

This process of fusion is mirrored in the frequent references to sun and light in the Helium proving. Moreover, descriptions of the 'the light of a million suns' are common in near-death experiences when the soul returns to its source.[14]

What then is the relationship between Hydrogen, Helium, and the death and incarnation cycle? While the description of sun and light appears in the Helium proving it does not feature in the Hydrogen proving. The proving of Hydrogen repeatedly describes a sensation of the soul leaving the body. One could speculate that the soul leaves the body as two 'hydrogen atoms'. During life these two were held together by oxygen in the form of H_2O, the water of life. As the dying body is deprived of oxygen, the mother molecule H_2O releases its two hydrogen captives. Thus the soul 'disintegrates' into its fragmented components at death. The two released soul fragments (H_2 or possibly 1H protons) finally reunite with their soul mate, four hydrogen nuclei fusing into helium. Thus at the end of the death process the light of a million suns appears. Here the Hydrogen journey ends and the Helium one begins, as collective soul fragments fuse into an

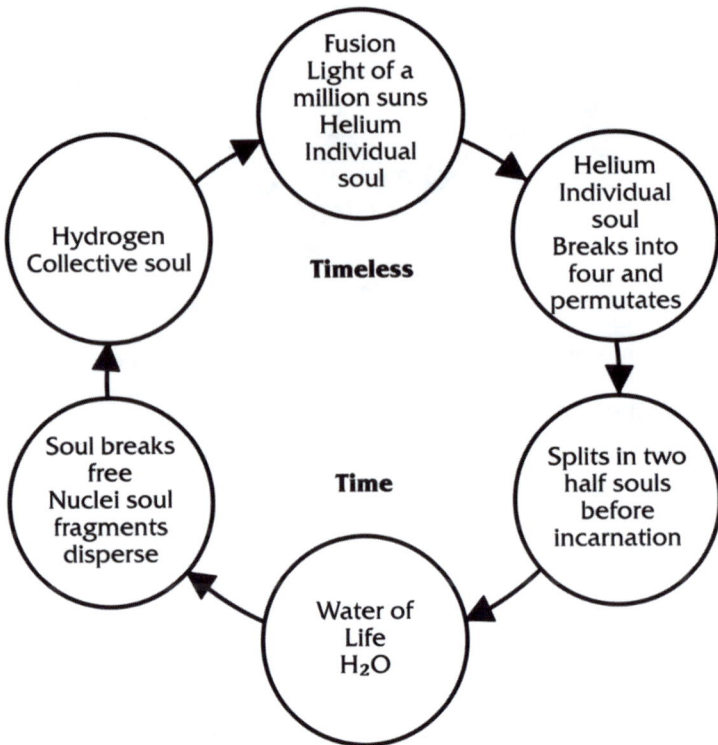

Figure 9.4 Cycle of soul and life

individual soul ready for the next incarnation. This moment, the time between death and reincarnation, holds within it all time and no-time. It is within this timeless moment that the 'journey of the soul' occurs, as related by Dr. Newton. See Figure 9.4.

Take us back through timeless state.

At the point of fusion, both hydrogen and helium share a state of undifferentiated oneness. As the Hydrogen fragments of universal soul fuse into Helium individual souls, the process of incarnation begins. At this point Helium is still a non-sexual, undivided soul, male and female united as one.

I woke and heard someone shout "Dad" and I responded as if they had shouted "Mum". I felt I was both or either.

The undifferentiated, non-sexual nature of Helium is also represented in the proving as a one-eyed person. One of my Helium patients had a dream of descending to earth on a unicycle, which is a similar idea.

Cabbala and the incarnation of the soul

As an introduction to the following sections it would be useful to get an idea of the process of incarnation according to the Midrash (Jewish Biblical interpretation) and the Cabbala. While many mythologies describe the journey of the soul as a direct one-step voyage from heaven to earth, the Cabbala contains a variety of descriptions of this process as a complex journey composed of multiple stages. The following is a synopsis of one of those versions, which has several parallels with our discussion of Helium.

The Midrash Rabbah says:[15]

> When the Holy One created Adam Ha-Rishon (First man – JS), it was androgynous. God created Adam Ha-Rishon double-faced, and split him/her so that there were two backs, one on this side and one on the other.

The Cabbalistic term for this is *Du-Partzufin* or "Double-Faced". These two faces or figures are arranged back to back (see Figure 9.5). The Midrash also states that Adam ha-Rishon was androgynous, being both male and female in one body, rather than hermaphroditic. Thus the soul begins its descent as an androgynous **double entity** composed of male and female. This means that at the highest stages there is absolutely no separation between male and female – all exists in complete unity. This idea of Adam having both masculine and feminine sides is found in the Midrash and the Talmud and is brought up in the context of reconciling the description of woman's creation which is found in the second chapter of Genesis, with the first description of the creation of Adam.

This stage is followed by a 'sawing of the two souls in half' known as *N'sirah*. This sawing relates to the biblical story in which a rib is removed

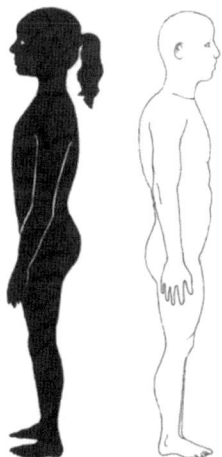

Figure 9.5 *Two faces, male and female joined at the back*

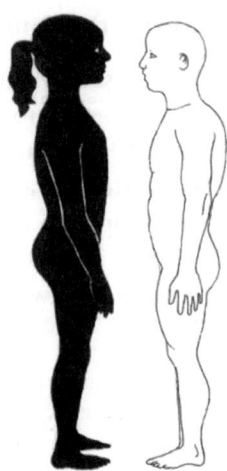

Figure 9.6 After being sawn apart the masculine and feminine turn to face each other

from Adam to create Eve. This particular rib is located in the back at the point where Adam and Eve are joined. Once they are sawn in half, they turn around to face each other (see Figure 9.6). From this point on, a love and sexual yearning for one another prevail.[15]

We are conditioned to think of Eve as having been created from Adam's rib. This is probably because most English Bibles follow the King James translation of the Hebrew phrase *achat mitzalotav* to mean "one of his ribs." However, it may also be translated as "one of his *sides*" i.e. one half of Adam.[16]

The significance of whether we translate the Hebrew *tzele* as rib or side is that the former implies that the feminine psyche per se did not exist prior to woman being assembled from a part of Adam. Whereas if we understand that God made Eve by dividing he androgynous Adam into two parts, the feminine Eve always existed together with her masculine counterpart in the original Adam.

One half of the 'sawn-in-half' souls descends into a waiting embryo and determines the gender of the person. The other half remains in the 'treasury of souls', ready to be assigned to another body.

The joining of two beings back to back is depicted in the myth of Janus. In Roman mythology, Janus was the god of gates and doorways, of beginnings and endings. He is most often depicted as having two faces or heads facing in opposite directions, though in earlier times he had four faces (see Figure 9.7). Often one face is shown bearded and the other one clean-shaven, in other words one is exposed and the other concealed.

The month of January is named after Janus, and the first of January was dedicated to him as representing a new beginning. The word janitor,

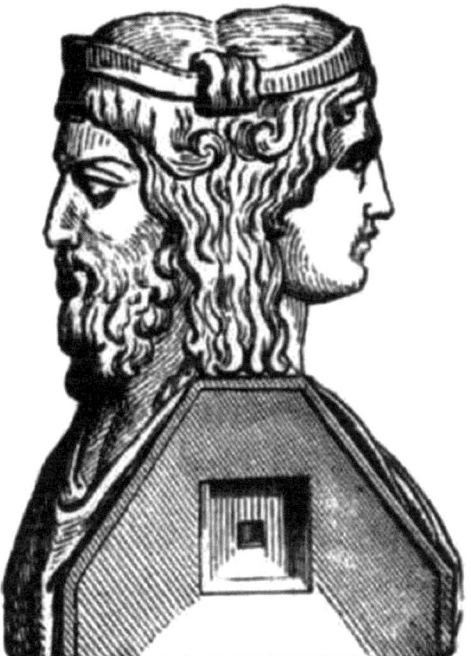

Figure 9.7 Janus, *the Roman God of beginnings and transitions*[17]

caretaker of doors and halls, also derives from Janus. In turn Janus probably originates from the Egyptian god Aker who was also seen as symbolic of the borders between each day, and so was originally depicted as a narrow strip of land (i.e. a horizon). He is depicted with heads on either side, facing away from one another, a symbol of borders. The Egyptians believed that the gates of the morning and evening were guarded by Aker.

Helium: Four into one, Nucleosynthesis of the soul

The fusion into helium actually requires six hydrogen atoms. Two hydrogen nuclei (protons) are left over at the end of the process. The net result is that it takes four hydrogen atoms to make one helium atom. We can theorise that six fragments of universal soul partake in the process of creating one individual soul, releasing energy in the form of heat, light and love. Two are left over (perhaps accompanying angels),[i] and four go on to

---

[i] In the bible the highest order of angels, the Seraphim, have six wings, while the lower order of cherubim have four Isaiah 6: 1–3, Ezekiel 1: 5–6.

make a new soul. As we will see this opens up the possibility of shuffling soul components to create a great variety of soul permutations. The infinite variety of individual souls (Helium) comes from combinations of these fragments of the original universal soul (Hydrogen).

In other words we all contain parts of each other's souls, which combine and recombine to create the diversity of life.

It should be noted that The Cabbala does mention that the soul is composed of many parts or sparks. Not all the soul parts will return to earth during each incarnation, but only those that need rectification.[18]

The analogy of the individual Helium soul being amalgamated from four Hydrogen atoms (nuclei) or universal soul fragments bears out well in the Helium proving. I initially believed that the Helium soul would consist of two entities, yin and yang, representing male and female energies.

However, the remarkable information gained from the proving is that the Helium soul is actually composed of four entities.

While Hydrogen has two basic particles, the yin and yang of proton and electron, Helium holds four particles. The following symptoms proves this point (see Appendix):

Dream about four men coming into my life. They were all very different from each other. I woke up with a feeling that a man is coming into my life, all of the four might suit me, not just 'the One'.

On the whole issue of destiny: Maybe we are squatters finding our double in another body? I have a sensation that I am looking out of another person's eyes with three other people.

The woman had two partners and this was her fourth child but who was the father? And also the thought there would be grandchildren to look after. Could I withdraw my offer and not take on someone else's responsibility?

The notion of a four-part soul is quite radical, as most esoteric traditions only consider one single, indivisible soul.

On further investigation of the four aspects of the soul according to Helium, the soul appears to be composed of a double male part and a double female part. The double male appears in the proving in a variety of forms: as two suns in the sky, as a double-ended penis and a sundog – a luminous ring or halo encircling the sun. Finally there appears a griffin: the lion and the eagle combined, both archetypal yang symbols.

Dream there were two Aryan men, both with large genitalia.

The wand/penis is double-ended, but one end is circumcised and the other is not.

Penetrating wands
Double-ended light
Expanding brilliance
Eternal sun.

These two male entities are not identical: One end of the double-ended penis is circumcised and the other is not (reminiscent of the Janus double image of two faces, one side bearded and one smooth). Thus we could describe the two different male forms as 'exposed male' and 'concealed male'. Another way to describe these two masculine energies would be 'male/yang' and 'male/yin'. In Chinese philosophy, yang represents the southern, exposed side of the hill, while yin is the northern, hidden side of the hill. Yang would be the front of the person, that which we usually see, while yin would be the hidden shadow that lies behind.[i]

Henceforth I will refer to exposed male/yang and to concealed male as male/yin.

As already mentioned, the proving also manifests two female entities, which I will henceforth refer to as 'female/yang ('exposed female') and female/yin ('concealed female'). In the proving this double female entity manifests in the following symptoms:

The great ambition of women is to inspire love – about double divine twins.

I was talking to two older girls in a young school, they needed partners?

I didn't know whether it was morning or afternoon, I had no concept of it because all was light. When I opened my eyes I saw the moon as if it were a second sun and the second sun arose in the east – it was the queen reflecting the brilliance of the king.

The Cabbala refers to the moon as originally being as large as the sun. The moon, which is essentially female, is now exposed in the bright light of the sun. In the following poem from the proving, we can perceive both the exposed and concealed female aspects.

Night in her reflected glory
Drawing back her cloak.
Revealing the stars
Guiding us home.
Solstice of darkness
Bearing the light.
Receptive is your womb

---

[i] This last aspect is opposite to the view taken by Traditional Chinese Medicine.

For receiving the light.
Vessel growing
In the watery darkness we float.
Hidden for a while
Before revealing our gift.
Receiving joyously
So we too may give.
All returns to the One.

As female/yin is both female and concealed energy, it is the most invisible aspect of the four-part soul, the 'dark side of the moon'.

Invisibility is apparent throughout Silvie's proving, together with a feeling of not existing. I remember Silvie telling me that she never had to buy a train ticket during this proving, the conductor just never saw her!

As if I don't exist. I had a delusion I was invisible to others but not invisible to myself.

I thought and felt transparent and beautiful inside.

I am trying to deny I exist.

Double withdrawal. Do I perceive the opposite all the time?

Seeing the invisible in the visible, and the indivisible in the one.

Soul permutations

Combinatory play seems to be the essential feature in productive thought.
Albert Einstein[19]

In the following sections I will discuss different permutations of the soul's four components as it evolves from the point of creation to final incarnation. It should be emphasised that nothing here is fact but merely a hypothetical analogy, a metaphysical game designed to show how a soul may unfold during the process of incarnation. Nevertheless this evolving sequence may be used to gain insight into the materia medica of Helium, the Biblical story, our relationship to God, others and ourselves.

In this section I will not discuss the various levels of spirit and soul as taught by the many other esoteric traditions, such as Egyptian, Tibetan, Rosicrucian etc. No doubt there are many interesting correspondences but I cannot cover them all. The information for these is readily available so that the reader may investigate and compare these paths according to personal preferences. The following ideas are based on the new information derived from the proving of Helium. I ask you to temporarily suspend what you already know.

Further symptoms related to this condition can be found in the Appendix.

As we have seen the complete Helium soul is composed or four entities:

Exposed male depicted as | Male/yang |

Concealed male depicted as | Male/yin |

Exposed female depicted as | Female/yang |

Concealed female depicted as | Female/yin |

First permutations

We begin with the first stage of total spirit, the primary soul combination. From all the possible combinations I have chosen the following to illustrate the initial sequence of soul evolution.

| Female/yin | | Male/yang | | Female/yang | | Male/yin |

I chose this sequence to represent the pre-heaven state (Ayin, no-thing or Tao) for several reasons. Most esoteric traditions (as well as information from the Hydrogen proving) talk of an initial, non-sexual, androgynous soul. Hence I have depicted the first sequence as alternate male and female fragments rather than a polarity of two male versus two female. Before creation and the contraction of God's light, both yins are on the outside, a reversal of the earthly norm in which yang is external. As in the Biblical story, before the beginning darkness lies on the face of the deep.

> Banished from home, night banishes the day.
> Night envelopes the day.
> Night cloaks the day.

As a result of this sequence, we find the light hidden deep within the dark, primordial chaos.

> Between the two.
> Towards BOHU.
> Dissolution.
> Shattered, scattered by the light.
> Shone, yet unable to create.
> Receiving, reassembling, unsure how to interact.

Bohu is a mystical word used in the biblical story of the first day: *Tohu va-Bohu* meaning the dark abyss of void.

Once God's light contracts from the centre, darkness or yin moves to the inside creating the void from which the universe will be born. Yang moves to the outside. The Big Bang is followed by hydrogen fusing into helium, creating light.

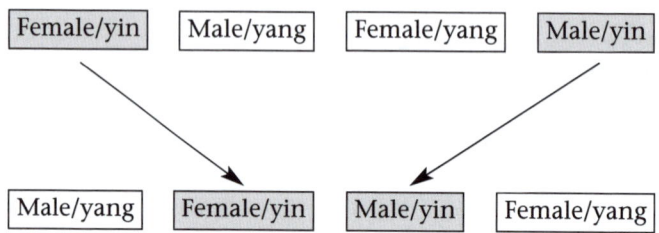

And God said: Let there be light, and there was light.

Day penetrates with light the night.
The queen is not dead, she is just not always seen due to the brilliance of the king.

This process is an involution of universe and soul. Light can be seen, while the middle void is concealed. As is the way of the material world, the yin root nourishes from the centre while yang expands to the periphery.

We now have a four-part, undifferentiated Helium soul composed of a pair of males entwined with a pair of females. Because of the alternate way the sexes are arranged (male/female/male/female) there is no left or right and no sexual charge. It may even seem as if we have two right sides next to each other. We could call these twin souls.

Sensation as if I don't exist. I felt as if I had a man inside of me. Filled in every way by a man.
Sensation in my right wrist that both sides felt the same. Was it left as well? Or inside out?

Because of the double nature of the soul at this point, the Helium proving features quite a few twins or doubles, people who appear in two places at once (cf. Appendix).

Second combination: Crossover

We now come across an intriguing and significant feature of the Helium proving: the crossover. As we transcend from spirit to matter the world inverts. We live through a mirror, reversing all we see with our eyes. Here are a few examples from the proving:

Dream: Crossing a road, looking after twins crossing the road to join each other. I joined many happy people walking in a line crosswise to meet us. I see self in everyone, in their own reflected image.

If two humans look into a mirror, do they see the same or opposite or reverse sides? Am I denying soul connections?

Enter the mirror, dive into watery reflection.

Wanted to shake hands with the wrong hand. This lasted all day

We will compare this crossover process to incarnation, meiosis, DNA replication and the Cabbala.

Soul crossover

As the soul descends into the body, it enters the first constriction point, the spiritual vortex or eighth chakra located directly above the vertex or crown chakra. This point is isolated at the tip of the 'wizard's hat' depicted in Figure 9.8.

I call it the emperor's chakra as I first learnt about it in the homeopathic proving of Jade. It is higher than the crown chakra, just as the emperor is superior to mere kings and queens. The emperor is undivided and symbolises the connection between heaven and earth, whereas kings and queens are divided and sexual, receiving their power from the people.

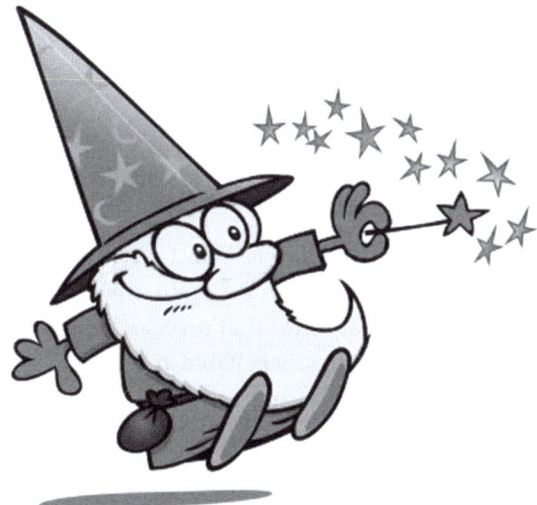

Figure 9.8 *The eighth emperor chakra is at the point of the wizard's hat*

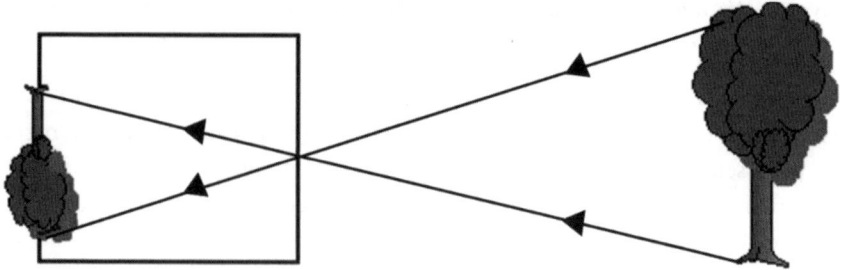

Figure 9.9 *A pinhole camera: The small opening causes the light to cross over*

When the soul passes through this narrow point, a crossover occurs, similar to when light flows through a pinhole camera (see Figure 9.9).

The result of this crossover is as follows:

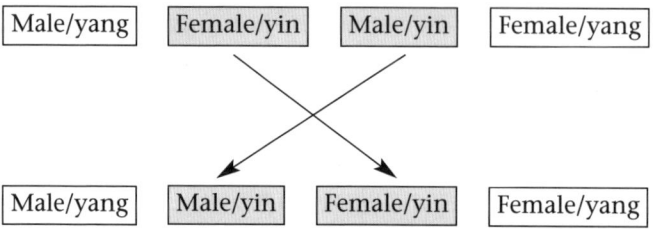

The male/yin and female/yin in the centre swap places. There are now two male quarters on one side and two females on the other, in other words the soul is now half male and half female. While the yang (front) sides are exposed, the yin (back) aspects are concealed. Here is the first Adam, composed of male and female facing back to back. This is the most transformative point of incarnation. We now have a four-part soul with a potential but as yet unmanifested sexual charge.

Cabbala crossover

In cabbalist terminology the crossover point occurs as we traverse the screen that separates the spiritual world from the physical world. This screen is also considered to be a mirror that reverses heavenly and terrestrial reality. One example of many is when Rabbi Joseph son of Rabbi Joshua dies and comes back to life. His father asks him: 'What did you see?' To which he answers: 'I saw a reversed world, the higher was lower and the lower was higher.' His father answered: 'You saw clearly, my son!'[20]

I wasn't sure if I was experiencing the opposite of everybody else or whether my interpretation was opposite. I wasn't sure whether it was everybody else or me, but I was experiencing the opposite of everybody else.

Experience was of opposites, yet memory of one.

Going in the opposite way, it was as if I was in another world, everyone was appearing so diverse and all men were appearing as one man.

I don't actually remember having a mother this time around. All these thoughts are fundamental. Do we search for the same or the opposite?

If two humans look into a mirror, do they see the same or opposite or reverse sides? Am I denying soul connections?

This reversal is also represented in the proving as the strange dream of walking backwards, one of the hallmarks of chronic disease. By living life through a mirror, we are always walking away from what we really need and towards what we imagine we want. This could be said to be the essence of chronic disease.

Dream: Recognising when people were unwell by the fact that they walked backwards.

Dream: On a bus with my mother going in the wrong direction.

The main consequence of this reversal is that the concepts of good and bad reverse. In the mirror image world of Psora we will learn to love what we hate and hate what we love.

Turn around

Up to this point, male and female are distinct but do not yet perceive their sexuality. The Cabbala states that Adam and Eve were initially joined back-to-back by one of their ribs. God then 'saws' them in half.

| Male/yang | Male/yin | Female/yin | Female/yang |

Sawed in half, becomes:

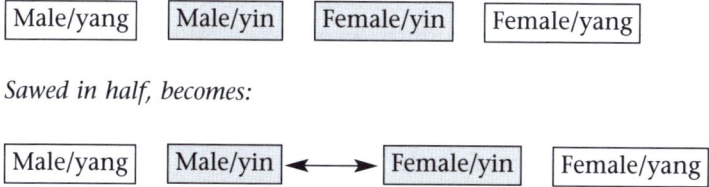

Once separated, they turn around to face each other.

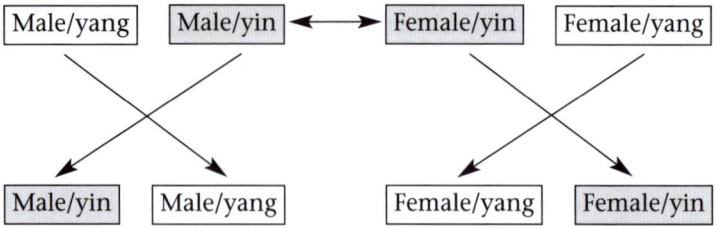

With this realisation I was female and not androgynous, like I had seen the masculine aspect.

It was the symbol of male and female union which could be used throughout life as polarity. Twins, looking at each other, joined, facing each other, union.

Light retreats back into the centre, eyes open. Adam and Eve 'see' each other's nakedness for the first time. They immediately feel shame and cover themselves up with fig leaves. Adam and Eve have eaten the apple. Knowledge is gained, truth is lost. And we get sex.

Sexuality

One of the main differences between the pre-crossover and the crossed-over soul is gender and sexuality. Hence the conflict of the 'pure' Helium soul who views the material, sexual world as a dirty and impure place. This aversion to sexuality is an important clinical indication.

Sex seems like a very gross way of communicating.

We come in one sex, unlike angels, so we need to connect with another.

Male and female – this is how it's done on earth. Until then you were androgynous, you didn't need sex. With that thought I was getting wave-like movements of the involuntary muscles of my vagina (multiple orgasm).

First Division: Male and female

The continuous, amorphous male and female sexual soul has just become aware of its sexuality. The two sides take a step back and cover up, thus dividing in two, one distinct male and one distinct female. The four-part soul now splits into two halves:

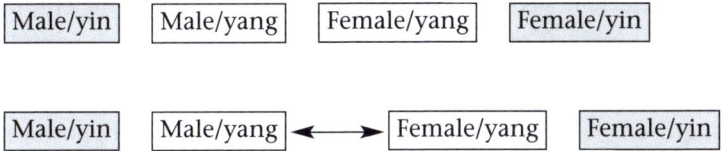

It feels like I am stepping from the oneness to the twoness.

The next stage of incarnation is the entrance of the soul into the physical body through the vertex or crown.

One half of the soul (two quarters) remains outside the body and one half enters as either a male or a female. In order to finally entre from spirit into body it must reverse polarities or change the direction of spin, like a screw being screwed inwards rather than outwards. If, as in the example below, a male is to be born it reverses direction and turns outwards. The other half that is not incarnating will stay in the same, spiritual, direction of spin.

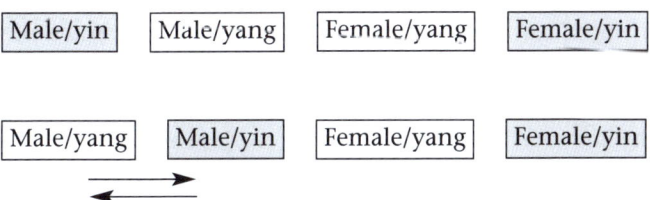

Until now the external aspects were either both yang or both yin, visible or invisible. For the first time in the sequence the external aspects are both yin and yang. Female spoons male. The sexes separate, let the war begin.

The end result of incarnation is therefore (For a man):

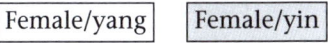

The remaining 'half soul' will either linger in a spiritual state or incarnate in another body, usually, but not always, one of the opposite sex:

Female/yang	Female/yin

These male and female halves are mirror images and represent soul mates, as opposed to the twin souls of the spiritual world. Their vital forces will spin in opposite directions.

I felt only half here yet functioning very well. I felt clear, efficient, light and calm, as if I had left my other half in a dream. Each half felt complete. Each half was very complete as a whole although it was a half.

You might be puzzled by me saying 'usually one of the opposite sex' above. It may happen that souls incarnate prematurely at various stages of the souls evolution and into an inappropriate body. I will not be addressing the complex gender issues that arise from these thoughts, as I wish to stay alive for a few more years. Work it out for yourself.

From this point on, the divided soul-mates will forever seek their sexual counterpart, yearning for completion. If they do not suffer too severely from psora and its consequent miasms, they stand a small chance of finding each other. Even if they do meet they may not always recognise each other, forever walking in the opposite direction away from their true goal.

Felt like no one would want to mirror me. Is our identity formed through the reflection of others?

I suppose it is about having the knowledge of love and seeing it draw away from you, out of reach somehow. But you have known it and touched it, and you know you cannot be the same any more. Once experienced, you cannot be whole without it and everything in your life seems incomplete without it. But even though it leaves its everlasting mark on you, it feels separate and apart from you. That causes great pain and sadness and I feel that now. Like the love of your life has gone out of your life and you will never be the same again, nor will the world around you. No doubt a similar feeling to man's fall from Eden.

Adam and Eve, the first manifested souls, live in the garden of Eden. Initially they are united as one person. Once they eat the forbidden fruit of knowledge, however, they differentiate good from bad, and separate into male and female. They are banished from the garden, which is guarded by an angel with a revolving sword, through which they (or we) cannot pass back again except through death or enlightenment. I think of this revolving sword as a mirror, one that prevents us from perceiving the true path home. Seeking our soul mate, the other half that will complete us, we approach this mirror. However, as we only see ourselves reflected in it, the reflection of our ego, we turn around and march in the opposite direction, doomed to the hopeless striving of chronic disease.

Second division: Front and back

As we saw in a previous section of the proving (Helium 10M), once the divided soul enters the body, one half (a quarter of the original soul) will migrate to the front of the eyes (yang, light) and the other half will recede to the hidden shadow side in the posterior (yin). See Figure 9.10.

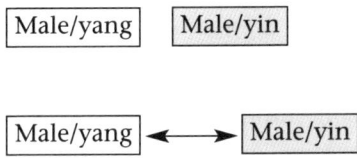

From this point on, the psoric person will believe he lives solely in the front of his eyes, identifying with one side of his personality. He will perceive and display the 'light' side, while the reverse 'shadow' side will appear in the guise of dreams, delusions, delirium, fevers, fears, swear words and sexual fantasy.

It is interesting to note that according to the noble gas provings, the migration to the front happens in two stages. While Helium drifts towards the eyes, the final stage of split belongs to Neon. Neon, which symbolises the birth process (*neon* meaning new), fixes the identity in the iris, finalising the split into front and back, light and shadow, and thus driving another

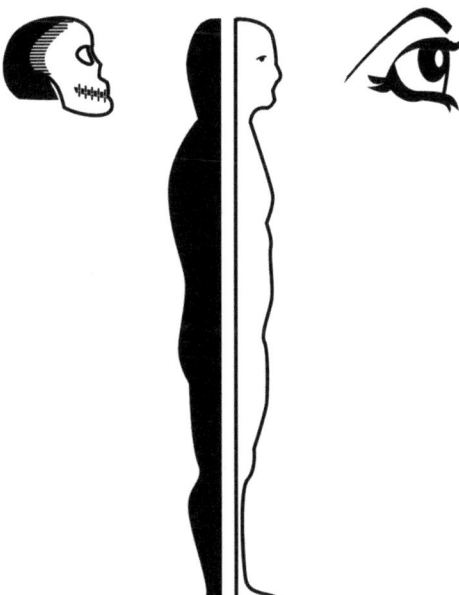

Figure 9.10 *Identification and shadow*

nail into the psoric coffin. We begin to believe what we see and that we are what we see. At the root of psora lies our fixed identification with only one aspect of our personality and humanity. Once we calcify a rigid sense of belief and identity into our ego, we lose flexibility, adaptability and, as a consequence, health.

In the morning dawns the opening of a radiant eye. I felt Neon was seeing the eye but Helium was seeing through the eye.

Helium proving

Image of being inside my iris and looking through. That is, I saw a large iris and I was looking through it. Light was radiating out from the centre of it.

Neon proving

I felt I was believing none of what I hear and only half of what I see.

Helium proving

The end result of this process is that every person has half a soul, and most live in the belief that their being is a quarter of the original souls (usually but not always the front half of the incarnated half soul). While the initial Helium soul was composed of four components, these have been 'reshuffled' through reverse, crossover and two consequent divisions. We may sum this concept up as follows:

Helium soul neucleosythesis: I am four in one

Neon post incarnation: I am one of four

In Edwin Abbot's book *Flatland*, the one dimensional line declares:[21]

Nature having herself ordained that every Man should wed two wives –" "Why two?" asked I. "You carry your affected simplicity too far," he cried. "How can there be a completely harmonious union without the combination of the Four in One, viz. the Bass and Tenor of the Man and the Soprano and Contralto of the two Women?

Graphic illustration

To make the concepts easier to understand, I have included a more continued illustrated progression (Figure 9.11). The following is the sequence of soul evolution from creation to total incarnation, with reference to the Biblical story.

Here is the sequence again, this time with human images, the four quarters of the soul. Front is yang, facing the light, and back is yin, the

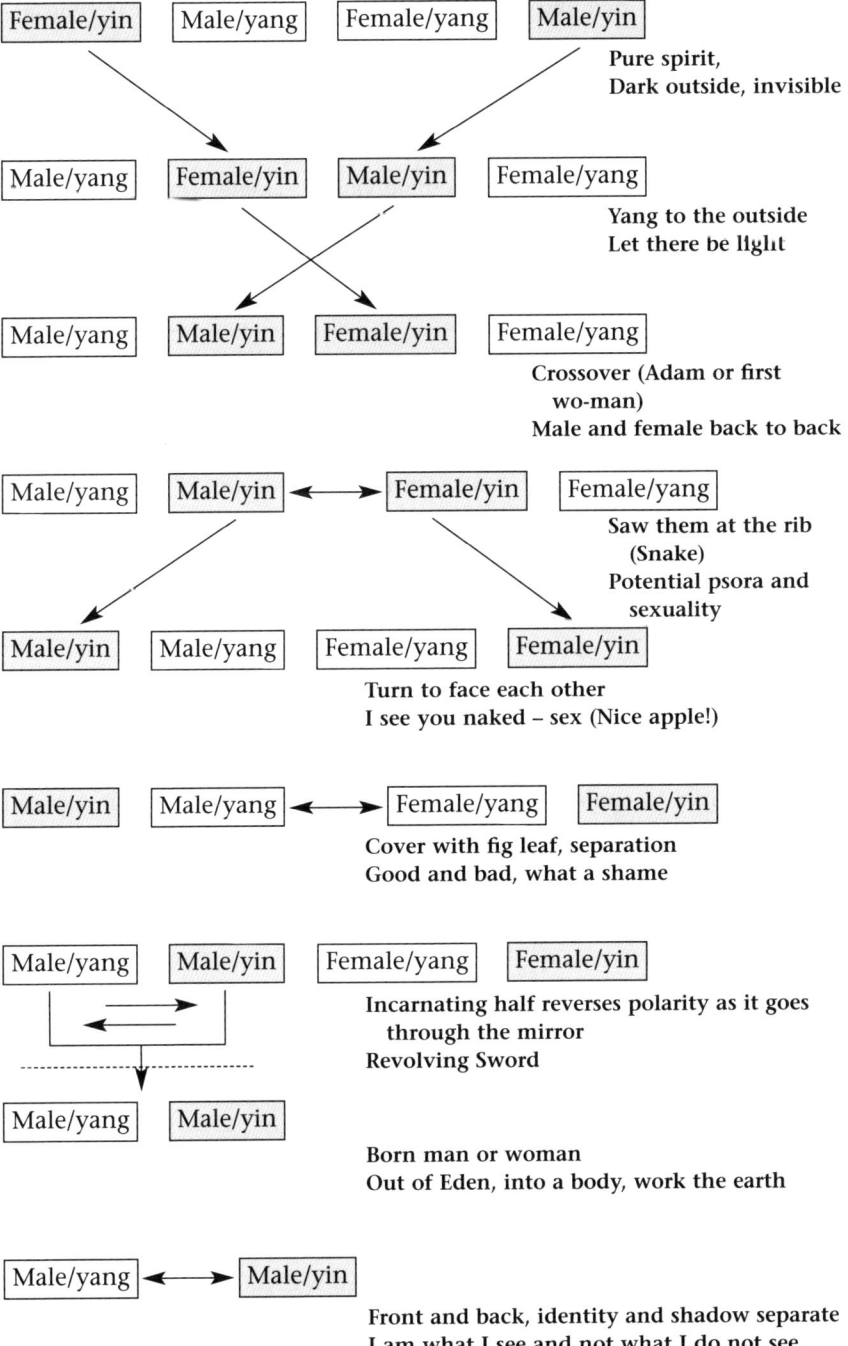

Figure 9.11 Graphic illustration of the sequence of soul evolution from creation to total incarnation

shadow side. The text illustrates possible patient expressions if they are 'stuck' in that stage.

In the first pre-heaven arrangement, the backs (yin) are on the exterior facing outside.

| Female/yin | Male/yang | Female/yang | Male/yin |

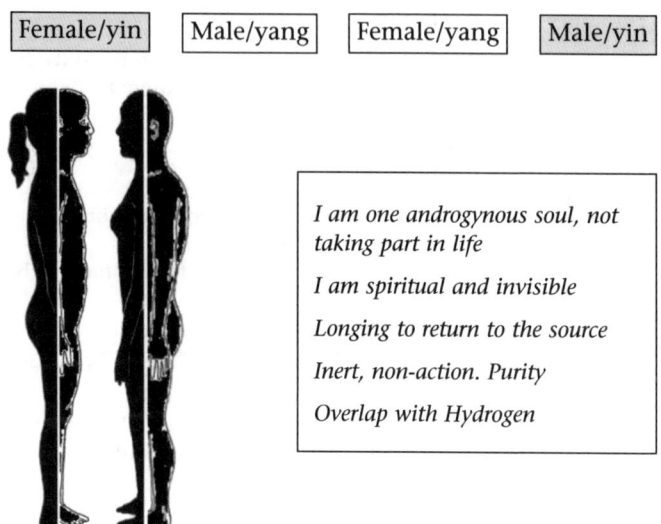

I am one androgynous soul, not taking part in life

I am spiritual and invisible

Longing to return to the source

Inert, non-action. Purity

Overlap with Hydrogen

Figure 9.12

Yang moves to the exterior. Light is created. Male and female are still mixed, thus they are twin souls.

| Male/yang | Female/yin | Male/yin | Female/yang |

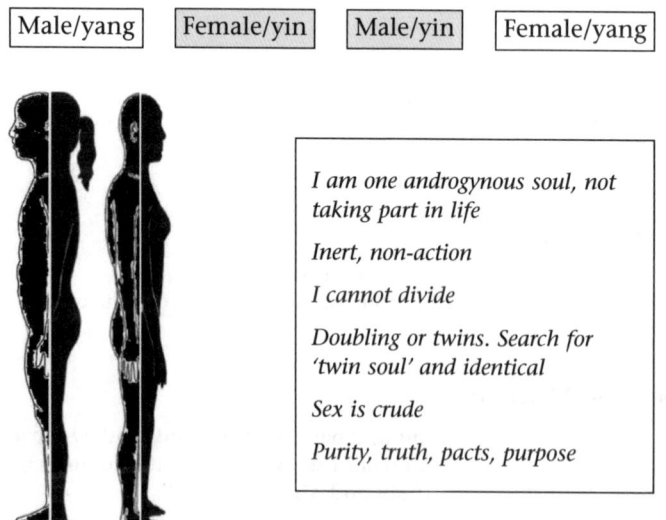

I am one androgynous soul, not taking part in life

Inert, non-action

I cannot divide

Doubling or twins. Search for 'twin soul' and identical

Sex is crude

Purity, truth, pacts, purpose

Figure 9.13

After the crossover the inner male and female change places resulting in a polarised sexuality. Truth reverses polarities in the mirror. They are now soul mates.

| Male/yang | Male/yin | Female/yin | Female/yang |

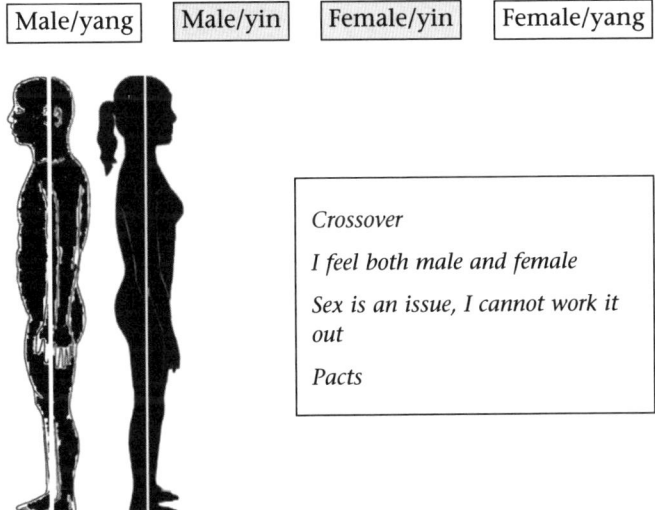

Crossover

I feel both male and female

Sex is an issue, I cannot work it out

Pacts

Figure 9.14

Adam and Eve are separated ('sawn apart') from the back rib. They turn to face each other, their eyes open and the see each other's nakedness. Knowledge is gained and truth is lost.

| Male/yin | Male/yang | Female/yang | Female/yin |

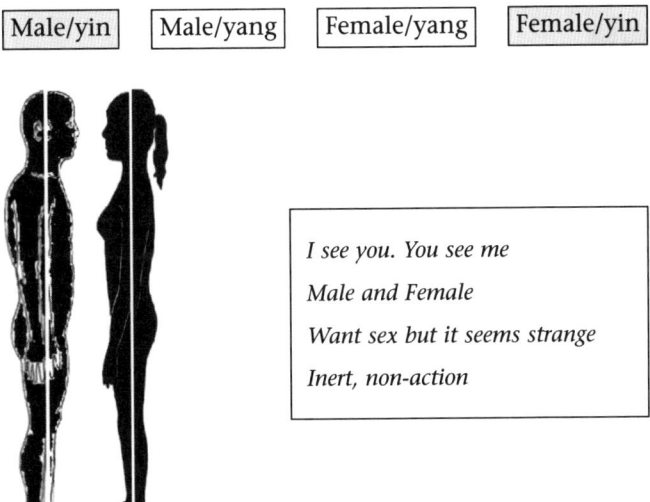

I see you. You see me

Male and Female

Want sex but it seems strange

Inert, non-action

Figure 9.15

Male–female separation occurs as they see each other and cover up.

| Male/yin | Male/yang | Female/yang | Female/yin |

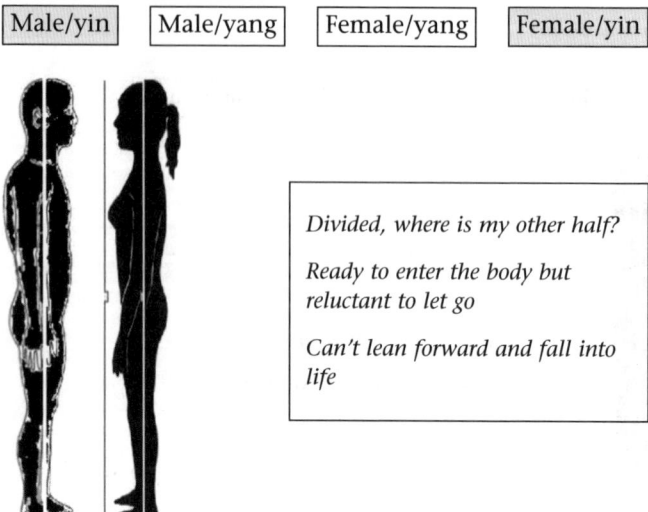

Divided, where is my other half?

Ready to enter the body but reluctant to let go

Can't lean forward and fall into life

Figure 9.16

Incarnation: Each half of the original soul, male or female, enters into separate bodies. Will they find each other? In order to come into the body the incarnating half must reverse polarities and direction of spin.

| Male/yang | Male/yin | Female/yang | Female/yin |

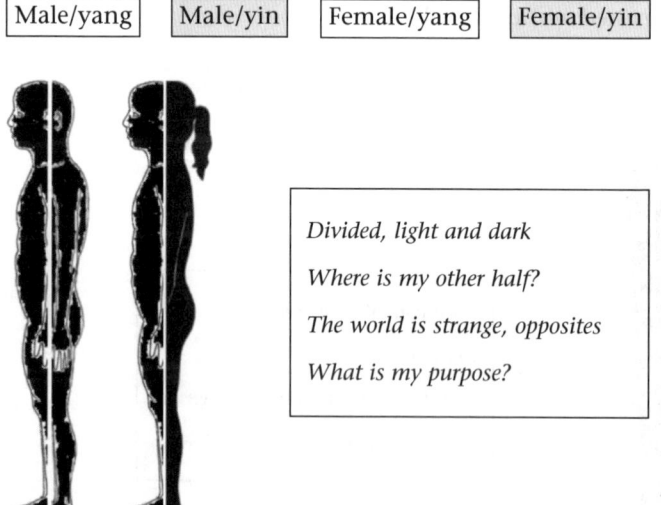

Divided, light and dark

Where is my other half?

The world is strange, opposites

What is my purpose?

Figure 9.17

Final split: Yang migrates forward and yin retreats into the shadow.

Male/yang   Male/yin

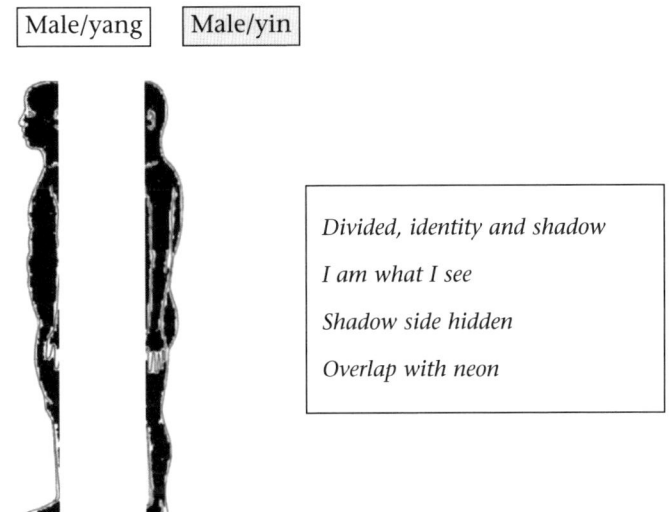

Divided, identity and shadow

I am what I see

Shadow side hidden

Overlap with neon

Figure 9.18

This concludes the permutation game. I am not able to supply prior references to all parts of my hypothesis, as it does not always accord with traditional views. I have wrestled with these sequences for years, arranging and rearranging them, and I am finally almost satisfied, though the mystery may never be fully solved. Naturally it is possible that reader's feedback will change my conclusions; I am open to that. I am aware that this theory may be right, wrong or irrelevant. I do however find comfort in some of the confirmations supplied by the analogies presented in the following sections.

The genetics of reproduction and incarnation

On studying the metaphorical model of soul incarnation as gleaned from the Helium proving, one is struck by the similarity to meiosis, sexual cell reproduction. Meiosis is the process by which male and female cells divide before sexual reproduction. During this process DNA **doubles, crosses over and divides**, resulting in **four** gametes which **then seek a mate** with which to recombine.

There are two processes by which cells divide: mitosis and meiosis. Mitosis is the normal development of cellular reproduction as it occurs in most body cells. Meiosis is the reproduction of sexual cells or gametes for the purpose of procreation.

Somatic cells divide through mitosis. During mitosis, the chromosomes duplicate and subsequently arrange themselves along the centre line of the cell. Both the chromosomes and the cell then split in half, resulting in two identical daughter cells. The genes on each pair of chromosomes match. These matching sets of chromosomes are known as homologous pairs, meaning they display the same genetic information.

Meiosis on the other hand is the division of diploid cells to form haploid cells or gametes. Gametes differ from somatic cells in that they only have half the number of chromosomes. During fertilisation, when the parent's sperm and egg unite, two haploid gametes fuse into a zygote, the first cell of a new individual. Half of the genes in the zygote come from the father and half from the mother. The number of chromosomes in this process is commonly expressed as $2n \rightarrow n \rightarrow 2n$.

Yet it is the only way 'back' to connect with the other. (1–2–1)

Reducing chromosomes from pairs to single copies is essential for successful reproduction, as it ensures that the number of chromosomes in an organism will not double in each new generation. Having even a single extra copy of a chromosome can result in serious complications. Down's Syndrome, for example, is the result of an extra copy of chromosome number 21.

Mitosis or asexual reproduction produces identical offspring and so allows both beneficial and negative characteristics to continue through the generations unchanged. Offspring produced by sexual reproduction, on the other hand, inherit an endless variety of combinations. The genetic diversity produced by sexual reproduction is the key to its power.

In some respects meiosis is similar to mitosis, yet there are fundamental differences. The primary difference is that two cell divisions occur in meiosis. Rather than the two cells produced by mitosis, there are **four** daughter cells at the end of meiosis, each containing one half of the chromosomes of the parent cell.

Meiosis is a complex process, which I will not elaborate in detail here. However a basic understanding is important for our comparison with the soul permutations of Helium. The following is an extremely simplified description of meiosis and is illustrated in Figure 9.19.

1   During cell division, each chromosome makes a complete copy of itself.
2   The copies, called chromatids, are linked by a centromere.
3   The homologous chromosomes line up.

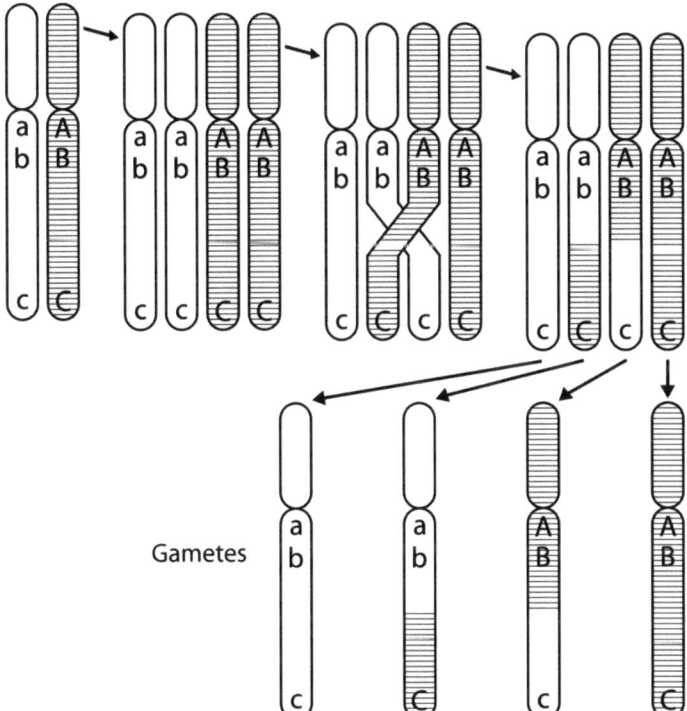

Crossing-over and recombination during meiosis

Figure 9.19 *The process of meiosis*

4   Crossing over occurs (in which two chromosomes swap male and female chromatid parts).
5   One of each pair of homologous chromosomes moves into a new cell (2 daughter cells are formed).
6   The chromatids separate and four cells are formed with a haploid number of chromosomes. These are gametes, sperm and ovum, ready for reproduction.

There are several parallels between meiosis and the evolution of the soul. The genetic material is **duplicated, two become four**, double yin and double yang. In the next stage, two chromosomes of a homologous pair exchange segments, producing variations of genetic material. This process is known as a **crossover**. As a result we get chromosomes with a mix of male and female characteristics. Finally there is a **splitting of pairs**, resulting in **four gamete** cells, each containing diversified genetic material.

The process of DNA splitting and copying itself is known as replication. Let us take a closer look at how DNA replication reflects in the proving. In

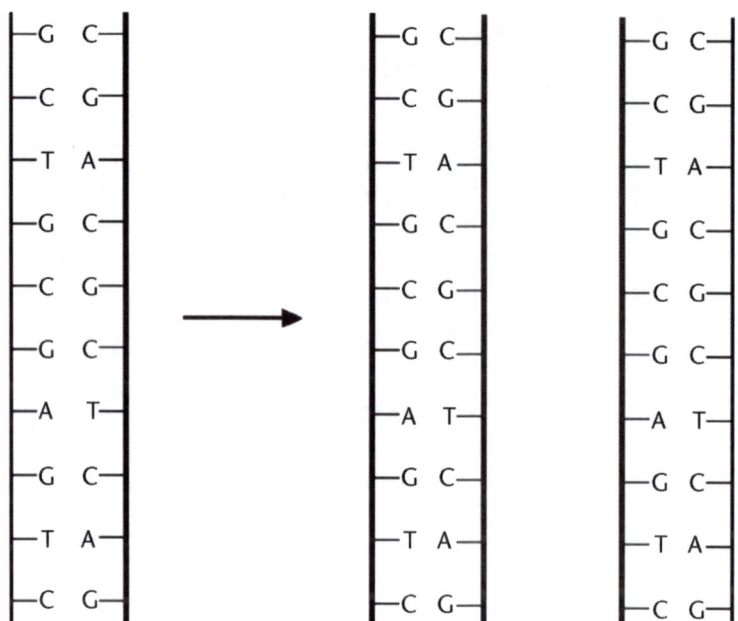

Figure 9.20 DNA replication

the beginning of replication the double helix unzips itself leaving two strands. Each strand is now a mirror image of the other. Using free-floating nucleotides, the strands now copy themselves into mirror images. Because A only bonds with T and C only bonds with G, both strands form exact matches. The two are identical.

Dream: A whole strip of stamps one below the other and the bottom row was ripped off.

Dream: On a bus with my mother going in the wrong direction. We both jumped off and I caught up with the number 11 bus at the junction. I looked down the left fork and the bus was down the right fork.

I was attracted to one of two young Asian men in the greengrocers. I felt the connection via a mirror.

Sunbeams (sun beams),
So we dance,
Spiralling together,
Tentatively at first,
Around each other.
Entwining then,
Touching yet,
How can this be?

Spirit soars,
Soul sings,
Together again,
At last,
As first.
In the beginning
There was one
Who became two.
Separated,
In order to multiply,
Returning to the one,
Go forth and multiply.

Both strands then cross over.

I have an image of a school sports team and choosing the sides you want to be on, and changing sides at the last minute as you realise you would in fact rather be on the other team.

Dream: I joined many happy people walking in a line crosswise to meet us. I see myself in everyone, in their own reflected image.

And divide.

I dreamt the coach was in two halves. I was on a single seat on the bus.

Both meiosis and the Helium soul progression relate to the very inception of life. The similarity between the two processes suggests that soul evolution shares a similar purpose to meiosis, namely **a shuffling of soul gametes to promote a diversity of incarnated souls**. If the incarnation process were similar to mitosis (as is generally supposed) we would all be the same over generations of incarnations. Clone souls producing a stasis of evolution.

There is, however, one serious logical flaw in this premise. Supposedly (but not definitely), each of the four soul fragments are identical to its entire brother or sisters fragments, i.e. all Female/yang soul fragments are similar. Since we are talking about four unchanging entities combining in a fixed series of patterns, the outcome will always be a fixed male/yin – male/yang or female/yang – female/yin. **There is no variety here**. All human incarnations would be the same, namely mitosis or a cloning of the souls. In order to uphold the similarity between Helium and meiosis, including its ultimate purpose of generating variety, I have had to expand this model. Enter soul DNA.

The soul as DNA

According to the principle 'as above so below' every spiritual essence has a physical counterpart. The closest physical equivalent to the soul is DNA. Located in the centre of each nucleus, DNA lends its inherent characteristics to the organism it inhabits, forming the material world in its image. The DNA molecule is a double helix, reminiscent of the souls spiralling journey through the labyrinth (see Figure 9.21).

Consider the following symptoms:

Image of spiralling downwards through lilacs and mauves.

Standing together, side by side, roots intertwining. Toe to toe, touch of hands.

The ivy puts you in touch with your own inner resources.

I felt the only way I could communicate was to lie down beside somebody.

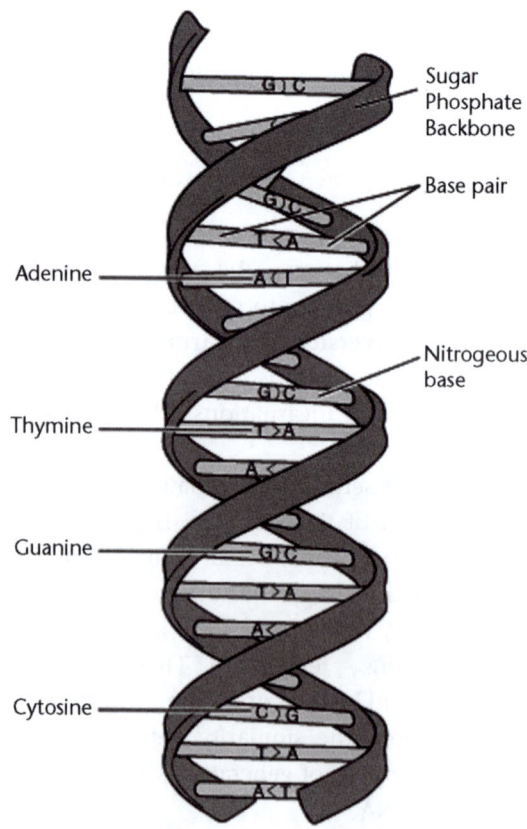

Figure 9.21 The double helix of DNA

A spiral maze. The spiral of the self and the search for self, symbolising the wandering of the soul circling inward and outward.

The dancing was all like this ((()))))((((0())). Like two sides of a circle, waiting for the other side. I looked across and saw a man, unpartnered. He started walking around towards me.

There is one other striking similarity. In our hypothesis, the soul is composed of four basic interchanging components. The same is true for DNA. Uniting the two strands of sugar phosphates that make up the double helix are four nucleotide bases: Cytosine, Guanine, Thymine and Adenine, (C, G, T, A). These connect in pairs through **hydrogen bonds** as C-G and T-A. Although the chemical building blocks of DNA are the same for every living organism, the sequence of these building blocks varies. The individual nature of each DNA strand is determined by the sequence of these four bases, which are arranged in triplets called codons, for example AGT, GCA or CCG (see Figure 9.22).

Because there are four possibilities for each base (C or G or T or A), each codon has 4 × 4 × 4 possible sequences, 64 in all. Each codon or sequence of three bases is a code for one amino acid. For example the codon AAA specifies the amino acid lysine and the codon CCC specifies the amino acid proline. At the moment there are 20 known amino acids in all. Similar to letters of the alphabet combining to form words, the order of amino acids dictates the final structure of the proteins which define our body. Proteins can be hundreds of amino acids long, so the possibilities are almost endless.

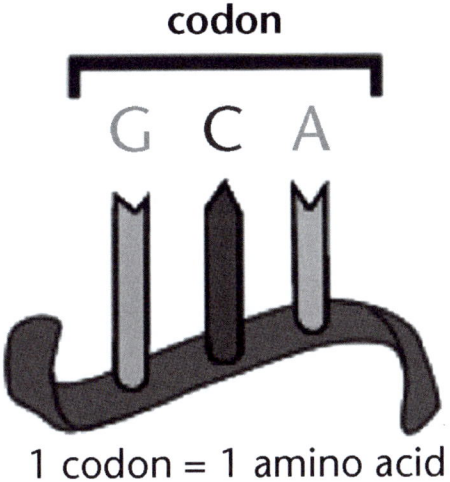

Figure 9.22 *A single GCA codon*

Dream: She is playing patience, laying the cards down quickly and deliberately in their sequences, deftly moving them around. I look at the cards. She is moving all the picture cards. I am very aware of the jacks, queens, kings, all the royals being moved about meaningfully.

As there are 64 possible codons, it is natural to compare these to the 64 hexagrams of the I-Ching. Note that there are various opinions on these relationships, which are beyond the scope of this book to discuss.[22,23] As an example, here is a Mandala illustrating possible correspondences between the many yin yang permutations and the codons. In the centre is the essential duality of life, yin and yang or Hydrogen. In the second ring, Helium, lie the four qualities of the soul or the four nucleotide bases: male/yang A (red) opposite female/yin T (blue) and female/yang G (white)

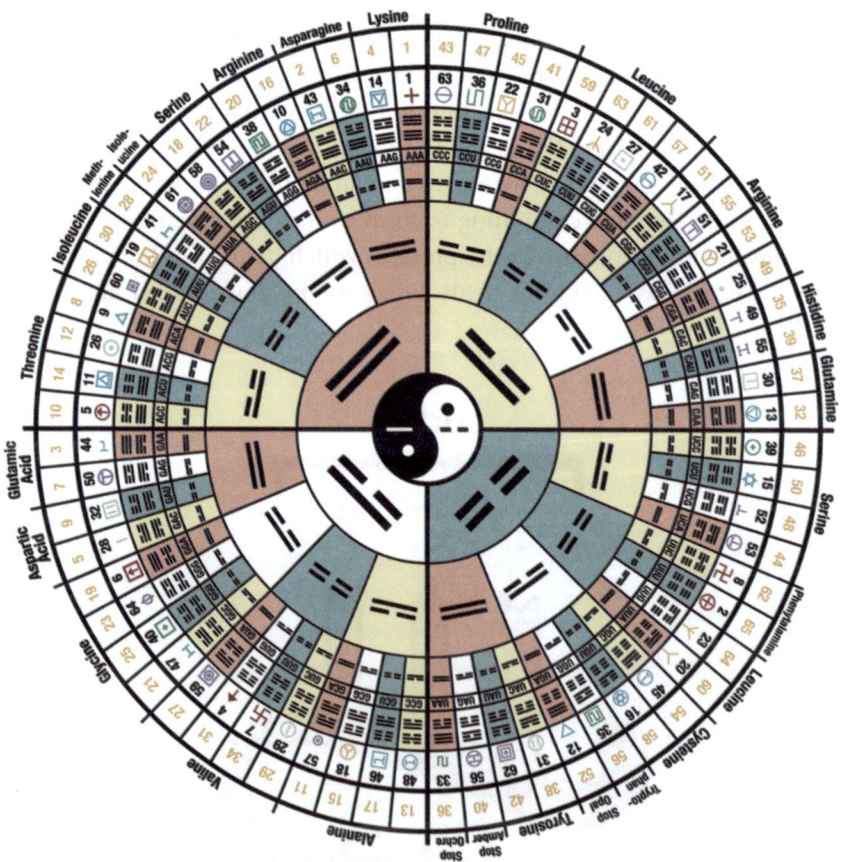

Figure 9.23 *Mandala illustrating the correspondences between the 64 possible codon sequences and the 64 hexagrams of the I-Ching.*[24]

opposite male/yin C (yellow). Each of these in combination with any of the other four gives sixteen possibilities in ring three. The final ring contains the 64 I-Ching hexagrams and the related codon sequences with the amino acids they produce.

We all go to the place where Tibetan monks are creating a sand mandala. The mandala was very beautiful and the colours were very bright and clear. It had been created from the centre outwards with infinite patience until it filled the whole square. One of the most fascinating things to watch was how the monks dealt with any mistakes. The misplaced grains of sand were gently and carefully moved to the right place with no sense of hurry or frustration. There was a great sense of patient acceptance and a sureness of purpose.

The following 'proving expression' puzzled me for a long time:

$2^5 = 32$

Note that rows six and seven of the periodic table consist of 32 elements each, 64 in all. These last two periods are the ultimate manifestation of nature's building blocks. They can be compared to the final two rings with 64 possible codon sequences. These codons generate the code for amino acids and proteins, the ultimate manifestation of our animal existence.

Using the DNA soul analogy, the four soul qualities correspond to the four bases A, C, G and T. Male/Yang would pair with female/yin and female/yang would pair with male/yin. These would arrange in a chain of soul codons whose sequence would dictate the essential blueprint of our being. Like the DNA molecule, each soul is actually composed of very many soul fragments arranged in a spiralling double helix. This would explain the huge variety of human souls, given only four soul fragments.

According to this idea, the arrangement of the four soul components is only one fractal of the double helix of our soul. Ultimately it is the combination of very many of these fractals arranged in sequence that decides our unique soul characteristics.

Like our individual soul, the communal soul of all humanity is arranged in chains of soul mates, families, groups and pacts, holograms of the purpose and structure of our collective existence.

Perhaps this analogy extends to Helium being suitable for genetically based disease. Time will tell.

Summary

Let us take a moment to summarise the metaphor. Photons are particles of light, corresponding to the cabbalistic term 'sparks' or fragments of God's light. At the inceptions of the universe, photons, together with other subatomic particles, form hydrogen atoms. Hydrogen atoms are analogous to fragments of the universal soul.

During death the soul departs from the body. This process appears in the Hydrogen proving but not in the Helium proving. It is possible that following death the soul disintegrates back into Hydrogen atoms, thus losing its unique individual identity. When the soul travels to the timeless place between lives it is no longer the individual soul that occupied the body, but instead fragments of the universal soul that were its constituents. Here they mix with other Hydrogen soul fragments in new configurations. The result of this process is that we are not the same soul incarnating repeatedly, but permutations of many soul fragments.

> Neither can I believe that the individual survives the death of his body, although feeble souls harbour such thoughts through fear or ridiculous egotisms.
>
> Albert Einstein[25]

As most religions and esoteric traditions refer to the same soul incarnating over and over again, this idea presents a new perspective. Of course many people have experienced what seems to be individual soul reincarnation or a past life experience, but it is possible that this is due to our identification with any one of the soul's fragments, who we erroneously consider to be our whole.

The conventional model of one soul incarnating time and time again in a 'cloning' or 'mitosis' mode does not explain the diversity of human life. Nor does it explain the strange rare and peculiar dreams that we experience. The Cabbala says that sleep is 1/60th of death, during which our soul partially leaves our body. During this mini-death we dream of an endless variety of morphing events and people in strange worlds that we would have difficulty imagining, and which may be explained by the interaction of our sleeping soul with the collective sea of soul fragments.

The recombining of soul fragments means we are composed of 'parts' of each other from different incarnations. It may be true that you were Cleopatra in a past life, but only a fragment of her is alive in you, rather than her whole soul. At the same time you might have a fragment of Xiao-Zien, a 16th century Chinese scholar, Henry the horse thief and an orphan girl from Africa who died at the age of two without anyone knowing she had ever existed. **Truly I am part of you and you are part of me.**

It may be possible that soul fragments interchange only within their soul group. **It is also likely that the lessons learnt are collective rather than merely individual ones**, and that the choice of which soul fragments combine with each other is a communal decision for the benefit of the whole group. If this is the case, healing only one member of the group will go a long way towards healing the whole group. Hence the ripples of true healing spread beyond the individual.

This remedy is about re-grouping into a group with people you really want to be with and who are really on the same path as you.

Michael Newton writes:[26]

The integrity of a soul's original cluster group remains intact in a timeless way. Regardless of who is graduating, they never lose their bond to old companions. Primary cluster groups began their existence together and remain closely associated through hundreds of incarnations.

When people in trance speak of being part of a soul cluster group, they are talking about a small primary unit of entities who have direct and frequent contact, such as we would see in a human family. Peer members have a sensitivity to each other which is far beyond our conception on Earth. . . . Members of the same cluster group are closely united for all eternity. These tightly-knit clusters are often composed of like-minded souls with common objectives which they continually work out with each other. Usually they choose lives together as relatives and close friends during their incarnations on Earth.

Naturally a hypnotised person will not be able to remember that in the world beyond he was but a fragment. From an earthly perspective this is inconceivable. We think of our soul as remaining whole in heaven.

During the process of incarnation, fragments of the universal soul reorganise and fuse into new combinations suitable for life's next lesson. Hydrogen fuses into helium. **By combining in infinite permutations in a similar way to the DNA molecule, these soul fragments create the diversity of the seven billion people living on this planet.**

The four types of soul fragments correspond to the four nucleotide bases. The process of incarnation is analogous to DNA replication in meiosis. The following is the journey of four soul fragments out of the millions that make up one soul DNA.

Four hydrogen soul fragments fuse into an individual Helium soul. Helium has no active role in the body. Its existence as an individual soul lasts only during the brief journey from spirit to matter, a timeless instant. The erroneous perception of a Helium patient is that he or she is stuck at any one of the incarnation stages: pure soul, crossover, doubles, twins, etc. This is a delusion because it is not the real 'here and now' of the patient.

At the first stage the Helium soul is not sexually oriented: double female intertwined with double male. These represent twin souls. The complete soul then enters through a narrow point where it crosses over and transforms into a potentially sexual yet undifferentiated soul. Subsequently the four-part soul is divided into two mirror images: soul mates. Each half will incarnate in a different womb unless they are twins, in which case they may incarnate in the same womb (it is possible that identical twins reincarnate at an earlier stage of the shuffle). Occasionally one half may remain 'in waiting' as a spirit, but I do not have the answer to whether, why or when this happens. Whatever the case may be, from this point onwards we are subject to loving, romantic and sexual yearning, constantly seeking our 'other half'.

At the end of this process half the soul or two Hydrogen soul fragments enter the body. Once in the body, the incarnated half will split again: One half (quarter of the original soul; gamete) migrates forward to become the external character, while the other half (quarter of the original soul) retreats to the posterior shadows. This final stage of this process is akin to the second period culminating in Neon. In the second period hydrogen combines with oxygen to create water or H_2O. Purely as a metaphor we could say that the two Hydrogen soul gametes are held together by oxygen as a water molecule, the fluid of life. When we breathe our last breath and oxygen is expelled as CO_2, it can no longer grasp the two Hydrogen soul fragments and they are released from the body.

The question that arises is: are all soul fragments of the same type identical? Are all the female/yang or male/yin fragments in the collective soul indistinguishable? If that were the case all memory of past lives would be erased. We know however that molecules retain echoes of their past, be they in mineral, vegetable or animal configuration. It should be acknowledged that as life develops into more advanced expressions it retains its past history and achievements. Photons, primary particles, atoms, molecules, cells, tissues, organs and organisms preserve something of their past nature, and achieved levels are sustained. (See the theory of process by Arthur Young.)[27]

Hence it seems possible that each soul fragment retains individual memories of its history, just as water retains the imprint of its source during potentisation, possibly through the unique configuration of hydrogen bonds or water clusters.

Dream: Packing to go back home. Going to the bus stop to catch the train with many others. In a hotel, a little girl ran off and I went to find her. She and I spotted my ex-husband perched on a tree that was hanging over the water, taking photos of the water or something in the water.

Regrouping

In a healthy non-psoric world, each person on earth would find their soul mate or even their twin soul. This would result in happiness and harmony on our planet.

Unfortunately, due to the nature of psora, the truth remains obscured behind a thin veil of deception, the 'mirror'. As a result most people tend to choose the wrong partners. Rather than our true love simillimum, we engage in similar, dissimilar, antipathic, allopathic or even inimical relationships. A recent study investigating pheromone compatibility showed that women taking the contraceptive pill tend to select unsuitable partners.[28] Here follows an example of such an 'inimical' choice, based on the analogy of inimical remedies.

Inimicals, as if

Inimicals as if
young miss Mercury
placed an ad in lonely hearts
for love and harmony.
She listed all her interests,
named her attributes
love of travel,
cinema,
eating foreign foods.
Her skill at bursting abscesses
and sweating from the feet,
a smile flashing caries
from rows of rotten teeth.
Her great aversion to the cold,
not to mention heat,
a tendency to ulcers
and making enemies.

Now Silica was smitten
when he read this ad
I've found the perfect partner,
I'm sure to make her glad.
She seems so similar to me
with foot sweats, ulcers and bad teeth,
restaurants and cinema,
aversion cold
and icy feet.
My, what a lovely pair we'll make
he mused while picking up the phone
I'll call her now,
we'll meet tonight,
who knows
I may just bring her home.

And so they met on their first date
with rising expectations
until the fan hit you know what
with little explanation.
For when they finally agreed
(it took an hour and a half)

on where to dine and what to eat
if you weren't crying
you would laugh.
She salivated on the food,
spread her butter thick,
he chewed his nails,
sipped some milk,
complained of feeling sick.
The movie was no better,
she opted for a thriller,
but when he saw the blood and gore
he promptly threw up dinner.
A short discussion followed
concerning music and pure tone
which ended in an argument
Mozart versus Rolling Stones.

And so the story goes
with Apis and Rhus-tox,
Calcarea and Baryta Carb,
Causticum and Phos.
The moral of this little tale
is plain for all to see:
A superficial match
will breed controversy.
Inimicals, as if.

Naturally finding a true soul mate is a blessing, but we make many mistakes along the way. These mistakes in our choice of partner are partly a result of combining according to the principle of the 'lower worlds'. In these worlds relationships or healing take place in accordance with the law of opposites known as antipathy, e.g. cooling a fever. Our search for a soul mate often results in lower level choices, perhaps based solely on one aspect of ourselves such as sexuality, which Hahnemann refers to as 'impure coition', the 'one-night stand of the soul'.

The ultimate choice of partner and relationship should be in accordance with the law of similars, the principle of the highest, most spiritual world. Relationships based on similars are a deeper matching of twin souls rather than the superficial matching of opposing soul mates prevalent in the lower worlds. The simillimum twin soul is elusive and can only be found once we become whole in ourselves. Mostly we would not recognise our twin soul if we saw hir (him-her). The union with our twin soul is in actual fact an inner reunion with our true self. So don't bother to go looking in the disco.

Shock of realisation, one divided, complete.

Luckily there are many levels of similarity approximating the ultimate union of twin souls. Just as 'the simillimum' is a theoretical concept which is nearly impossible to achieve in practice[29] finding our soul mate and ultimately our twin soul is a long learning and healing process that takes many lifetimes. It is the power of similars that guides us on our convoluted journey back to oneness. In the meantime as the song says, 'If you can't be with the one you love, love the one you're with'.

Simillimum, as if

Similimum as if
only one bulls eye,
an all or nothing contest,
be perfect or don't try.

As if three thousand arrows,
could cure a million men,
but if they miss,
then no result,
we have to shoot again.

When climbing up the mountain,
towards a single peak,
many sights along the path,
cause the heart to sing.

In theory every soul,
has one analogy,
but when it comes to love
let's face reality.

Soul mate, stranger, lover, friend,
acquaintance or brief meeting,
inimicals or follow well
not always what we're seeking.

Many people cross our path,
each a remedy,
we seek that one connection,
the one to set us free.

Some day true love comes to all,
but in the brief meanwhile,
why not have a sweet romance,
with your close simile?

And please be gentle with yourself,
when your best endeavour,
touches the periphery,
but doesn't last forever.

Simillimum, as if.

Our progress or regression in life's evolution depends on the similarity of our choices, be it partners, relationships, spiritual masters, professions, friends, home or even body. Poor choices compound over the generations, creating a chaotic state of unhappiness, conflict and disease, the flowering of psora. As we grow healthier, however, we are more likely to make more appropriate and similar choices, thus rectifying our lives. Through proper living and healing, we clean the coating of prejudice from the lens of our mind. With every right action we create possibilities for more right actions, with every purification of body, mind and spirit we perceive the world around us more clearly. As a consequence, we are more likely to select a partner approximating our simillimum. This unification then leads to further healing, ultimately evolving the human race as a whole towards the eradication of psora.

Choices

Every act of strength leads to another act of strength
Every act of weakness leads to another act of weakness
Courage begets courage
Fear breeds fear.

Kindness multiplies
Small acts generate small acts
Big acts generate bigger acts
Humour infects.

Desire spawns need
Need decays to dependency, addiction.
Facing pain and overcoming difficulty
Enhance freedom and power

Respect empowers.
The essence of respect is
Listening,
Truly being
Other points of view.

Life spirals up and down
Snakes and ladders.
At every moment,
Choose your path.

Once decided, don't look back
Move on. Gateways will open.
At all times
the universe is unfolding as it should.

With each homeopathic relationship of soul or remedy we are healing ourselves and the world around us. Soul mate to soul mate, twin soul to twin soul, group to group. Gradually we enlarge our limited concept of truth towards the greater truth. Each fragment of universal soul that finds its mate or receives a similar remedy helps to rectify other members of the group. Each soul correction goes a long way towards healing the collective.

The human DNA molecule contains around three billon nucleotide pairs. Extending our analogy to a wider perspective, we might say that the DNA molecule represents the whole of humanity, in which each soul is just one codon: four bases, three pairs, 64 combinations. This blueprint has been scrambled over the generations, the result of countless poor choices. To recreate the image of the perfect being, we must restore the collective soul DNA to its original sequence. This includes relationships between lovers, family, friends, neighbours, teachers, pupils, professions, spiritual practices and home locations.

According to the Cabbala, the fragmentation and scattering of the light into countless sparks has a purpose.[30] Through this journey the singular, all-pervading light of God is transformed into a multitude of unique living beings, bestowing beauty and diversity on the world, along with the opportunity for learning, evolution and rectification. The final objective of creation is 'Tikun' or 'the end of correction', rearranging the sparks in the original sequence so that universal harmony will prevail. This amalgamated humanity is termed Adam Kadmon, meaning the 'Original Adam'. The main characteristic of this stage is that what is true for any one individual is true for the whole of humanity and vice versa.

The homeopathic idiom *'as if one person'* applies to epidemics and miasms and well as to individuals. It represents a state of disease because of the delusional nature of the term *'as if'*. A healthy person should be *'one person'* with no *'as if'* attached. In a similar way, healthy humanity should live as one person in harmonic resonance rather than in fragmented conflict. We should all be subject to one universal truth, rather than our splintered versions of it.

This idea is reflected in what is arguably the most important word of the most important sentence in the most important paragraph of Hahnemann's *Organon*, §9

Towards the higher purpose of our existence.

Paragraph nine of the *Organon* represents the ultimate destination of health and cure. As such it is the peak of the entire *Organon*. It is the physician's mission to restore the sick to health, and these seven words express the reason for this health, the purpose of all our endeavours. At the very core of this sentence is the word 'our', the axis around which the entire *Organon* revolves. If we were to replace '*our*'; with '*my*' the whole meaning of the paragraph and consequently the entire *Organon* would change. Health would become a self-centred endeavour, and our work would generate nothing but egotism and greed. We would continue to exist '*as if*' one person rather than to actually live as one person. Our collective mission is the progression from 'my' to 'our', reuniting soul fragments in their original sequence, back into the collective Hydrogen soul and beyond, to the source of all souls, the One.

> Strange is our situation here on earth. Each of us comes for a short visit, not knowing why, yet sometimes seeming to divine a purpose. From the standpoint of daily life, however, there is one thing we do know: that man is here for the sake of other men, above all for those upon whose smiles and well-being our own happiness depends.
>
> Albert Einstein[31]

References

1 Seelig C. *Albert Einstein: a documentary biography*. London: Staples Press; 1956, p. 194.

2 Einstein A. Religion and Science. *New York Times Magazine*. November 9th 1930 pp 1–4. Available online at: http://tinyurl.com/8zdl

3 Schwartz H. *How the Ari Created a Myth and Transformed Judaism*. Tikkun website. Available online at: http://tinyurl.com/7jm3b2z

4 Vital C. Etz Chayim, 11b. In: Ariel DS. *Mystic Quest: An introduction to Jewish Mysticism*. New York NY: Schocken Books; 1992.

5 Lao-Tsu *Tao Te Ching* (Feng G-F, English J, Lippe T. trans.), New York NY: Random House/Vintage Books; 2011. Chapter 23 Available as Kindle edition and also online at: www.questia.com/Online_Library

6 Eising N. *The Proving of Vacuum*. Kileenora, Co Clare: Burren School of Homeopathy; 2000.

7 Matt DC. *God & the Big Bang: Discovering Harmony Between Science & Spirituality*. Woodstock VT: Jewish Lights Publishing. 2000.

8 'As above, so below.' The Mystica. An on-line encyclopedia of the occult, mysticism, magic, paranormal and more... Available online at: http://www.themystica.com/mystica/default.html

9 How the beginning created God – Elohim. In: Blaha J. *Lessons from the Kabbalah and Jewish History*. Brno Cz: Mark Konecny; 2010. Chapter iii: The Zuhar and the Lurianic Kabbalah. p. 118. Available online at: http://tinyurl.com/84p2e8l

10 Leet L. *The Secret Doctrines of the Kabbalah*. Rochester VT: Inner Traditions International; 1999.

11 Hanson K. The Age of Enlightenment. In: *The Untold Story of the Mystic Tradition*. Tulsa OK: Council Oak Books; 2004. p. 152.

12 Hahnemann CFS. *Oragnon of Rational Medicine*, 6th edition. (Dudgeon RE trans.) Philadelphia PA: Boericke and Tafel; 1896.

13 Sherr J. 'Paragraph 103' *The Homeopath* 2010; Spring. Northampton: Society of Homeopaths.

14 Atwater PMH. *The big book of near-death experiences: the ultimate guide to what happens when we die.* Charlottesville, VA: Hampton Roads Publishing; 2007.

15 Midrash Rabbah, Bereshit 8:1 For more information see http://neohasid.org/kabbalah/creation/

16 Matt DC. *Zohar: Annotated & Explained.* Woodstock VT: Skylight Paths Publishing; 2004.

17 http://hifranchise.files.wordpress.com/2011/01/janus-clipart.jpg

18 Sha'ar ha Gilgulim (Gate of Reincarnations, Rabbi Chaim Vital, based on the teachings of the Arizal, Rabbi Rabbi Isaac Luria Zohar in Parashat Mishpatim.

19 Einstein A. From a letter to the French Mathmetician Jacques Hadamard written in 1945. In: Hadamard J. *The Psychology of Invention in the Mathematical Field.* Mineola NY: Dover Publications; 1954.

20 Talmud, Baba Batra 10; 2.

21 Abbott EA. *Flatland: A Romance of Many Dimensions. 1884.* Amazon CreateSpace Independent Publishing Platform 2013. Available online at: http://tinyurl.com/68km5t

22 Schonberger M. *I Ching and the Genetic Code: The Hidden Key to Life.* Sante Fe NM: Aurora Press; 1992.

23 Yan J. *DNA and the I Ching: The Tao of Life.* Berkeley CA: North Atlantic Books; 1993.

24 The Abysmal website http://tinyurl.com/cn8foop

25 Einstein A. *The World As I See It.* Secaucus NJ: Citadel Press; 2000.

26 Newton M, Journey of Souls – Case Studies of Life between Lives Woodbury MN: Llewellyn Publications; 1994. See also http://tinyurl.com/7o8sl3n

27 Young Am. *The Theory of Process.* See http://tinyurl.com/7xkw26f

28 Anon. Contraceptive pill 'can lead women to choose wrong partner'. *The Guardian* 13 August 2008. Available online at: http://tinyurl.com/dbkx4c

29 Hahnemann CFS. *Oragnon of Rational Medicine*, 6th edition (Dudgeon RE (trans.) Philadelphia PA: Boericke and Tafel; 1896. §156.

30 Robinson G. Isaac Luria and Kabbalah in Safed. My Jewish Learning Website. Available online at: http://tinyurl.com/72x43x2

31 Einstein A. In: *Living Philosophies* New York NY: Simon and Schuster; 1931. Available online at Science and Philosophy website: http://tinyurl.com/87fwdqd

10

FURTHER ANALOGIES

Four in one

The four qualities of the soul may be compared to the four initial forces of physics: electromagnetism, gravity, strong and weak. The comparison is based on the premise that both soul components and basic forces are energetic building blocks of the universe. The following is merely suggestive:

TABLE 10.1 The four universal forces and correspondences

Electromagnetic	Infinite range	Electricity, magnetism and light	Male/Yang
Gravity	Infinite range	Force acts between all *masses*	Female/Yang
Strong	Short range	Binds *neutrons* and *protons* together in the cores of atoms	Male/Yin
Weak	Short range	Beta decay (the conversion of a neutron to a proton, an *electron* and an antineutrino)	Female/Yin

Like the universal forces, the four elements of fire (male/yang) air (female/yin) earth (female/yang) and water (male/yin) may also represent four part nature of the soul. We can also compare the four universal soul fragments to the four human blood types: A, B, AB and O. Type O blood, combining with any of the other types, is comparable to female/yin, the most receptive of the four fragments. Blood type AB, combining only with itself, would represent the extroverted masculine male/yang soul gamete.

The hearts' chambers are another mirror to the four aspects of the soul. The left and right side represent male and female, each with a receiving yin atria and pumping yang ventricle.

Jewish mystical tradition contains many references to four basic qualities. The Bible tells of a single river flowing through the garden of Eden, which represents the unity of the divine soul. Once this river leaves the garden, it splits into four heads representing diversity. Four Archangels are mentioned in the Cabbala: Michael, Gabriel, Uriel and Raphael. The *Mishna* (early Jewish interpretations of the Bible) mentions four sons: One wise, one wicked, one naïve and one who is too shy to ask. Jerusalem is divided into four quarters which are said to be analogous to the four chambers of the heart. The Tree of Life exists in the four worlds of the creation, namely Atziluth, Briah, Yetzirah, and Assiah, representing the descent from pure spirit into matter.

The Cabbala abounds with examples of one divided into four emanations. Here is one instance:

> You should also know that it is exactly the same with all the ten sefirot of each and every world. . . . Every higher aspect is called Emanator relative to the aspect lower than it, which is called emanated. And the **emanated is always divisible into four letters,** even in any one of its ten sefirot, or in any one of the ten sefirot of any one of them. . . . Understand this well; it is a key to understanding all the lessons.[1]

Perhaps the most striking correspondence to the four aspects of the Helium soul is the book of Ezekiel, which is most specific about four angels with four faces and four wings each. Two wings are open and two closed. There are four faces; man, eagle, lion and ox. The following emphases are mine:

> And I looked, and, behold, a stormy wind came out of the north, a great cloud, with a **fire flashing up,** so that a **brightness** was round about it; and out of the midst thereof as the colour of electrum, out of the midst of the fire. And out of the midst thereof came the likeness of **four living creatures.** And this was their appearance: they had the **likeness of a man.** And every one had **four faces,** and every one of them had **four wings.** And their feet were straight feet; and the sole of their feet was like the sole of a calf's foot; and they sparkled like the colour of burnished brass. And they had the hands of a man under their wings on their **four sides;** and as for the faces and wings of them four, their **wings were joined one to another;** they turned not when they went; they went every one straight forward. As for the likeness of their faces, they had the face of a man; and they four had the face of a lion on the right side; and they four had the face of an ox on the left side; they four had also the face of an eagle. Thus were their faces; and their wings were stretched upward; **two wings of every one were joined one to another, and two covered their bodies.**[2]

Finally, the city of Hebron is mentioned in the proving.

I was hoping there would be peace in Hebron.

Hebron is the town called the **city of four** (*kiryat arba*). It contains the cave of Machpela (literally meaning 'the doubling cave'), which is said to be the gateway to heaven. Abraham paid 400 shekels for the site. Four couples are said to be buried there: Adam and Eve, Abraham and Sarah, Isaac and Rebecca, Jacob and Leah. The Zohar has a lengthy discussion on the arrangement in which they were buried and the various possible permutations of this order.

Twins and Doubles

Twins feature very prominently in the proving.

I felt I was seeing the twin of everything but not seeing double. It was the twin.

I am travelling on a train and two seats in front of me I see a pair of twins and am fascinated by them.

Dream: Crossing a road, looking after twins crossing over a road to join the other.

Fraternal twins develop from two separate eggs that have been fertilised by two separate sperm. Identical twins develop from a single fertilised egg (zygote). In the latter case, at a relatively early stage in its growth the zygote splits into two separate cell masses which go on to become embryos. These embryos are genetically identical to each other and are always of the same sex.

It may be that twins are related to the soul before the first division into two. At this stage we have twin souls, a non-sexual affinity. While identical twins and doubles would be analogous to mitosis of the soul, non-identical twins would be associated with meiosis.

A curious experience in the proving is that of doubles, identical people seeming to appear in two places at once. This strange phenomenon happened to several people during the proving, one reporting that she saw me or an exact replica of me in a place I had never been before. Another prover states:

I saw somebody who couldn't possibly have been there. It was their double and they were there, but I knew it was impossible.

Provings can only manifest phenomena that exist on some level, so if a prover observes doubles we can assume it is essentially possible for a person to appear in two places at once. Dr Newton speaks of a single soul incarnating in two places at once (to gain double the experience).

The idea of doubles appears in several anthropological texts as well as in the Cabbala. The soul, which partly incarnates and partly remains as an energetic body, can remanifest in different places at once. This phenomenon was discussed by Sigmund Freud in his essay 'The Uncanny'. A Viennese physician and poet by the name of Schnitzler referred to Freud as his "double", while Freud called Schnitzler his "psychic twin".

Theosophy

According to theories popularised by theosophy and in a modified form by Edgar Cayce, God created androgynous souls, which are equally male and female. The souls subsequently split into separate genders. Over countless reincarnations, each half seeks the other. When all karmic debt is purged, the two will fuse back together and return to the ultimate.

Twin flames are very different and very rare. Twin flames are two people in two separate bodies that share the same soul. Twin flames meet each other in their first incarnation so they remember the soul frequency of the other being. They are usually reunited during their final time on this planet. If twin flames meet before they are ready, they can be total opposites and not at all compatible. When twin flames meet and are ready for each other, it is the most enjoyable experience possible on earth. At this point, twin flames are almost identical. They truly complement each other and it is a hardship for them to be apart. As an outside observer it is sometimes hard to tell the two people apart. They have a very strong bond and often experience telepathy with each other. Their lives often have many parallels, even before meeting each other. Again, meeting your twin flame is very rare on this planet.

Moses

As we will see when we progress through the noble gases, each is related to one or more noble figures, the 'superheroes' of history and mythology.

Moses started the first monotheistic religion in the world, the belief that God is one. According to Jewish lore, Moses is the only person ever to see God face to face. He climbs to the top of Mount Sinai, which is covered in smoke and flame, where he talks directly to God. This is a return to a Hydrogen state. He receives two stone tablets, Hydrogen's one fused into Helium's two. On the two stones are inscribed the Ten Commandments:

Helium, element two, heralding Neon, element ten. These commandments are the rules of life which Neon will need in order to conquer its desires. When Moses descends the mountain his face is shining. But the Israelites have substituted the golden calf (Aurum) for God's light (Hydrogen).

After a long journey in the wilderness Moses is not allowed into the land of Israel. It is said that this is due to Moses using a staff rather than 'the word' to split the rock and obtain water. Like a soul that cannot enter the body, he views the holy land from the top of Mount Nevo, yet cannot enter it.

Alchemical stage

According to the hermetic tradition there are seven alchemical stages in the process of physical and spiritual transformation and transmutation. The first of these is Calcination.[3]

Chemically, the Calcination process involves heating a substance in a crucible or over an open flame until it is reduced to ashes.

On a spiritual level Calcination is the destruction of ego. Calcination helps us to find our true self by removing layers of false persona, identifications, illusions and attachments to worldly goods. To attain this purification the ego must be "burnt" before it can be reconstructed in a way

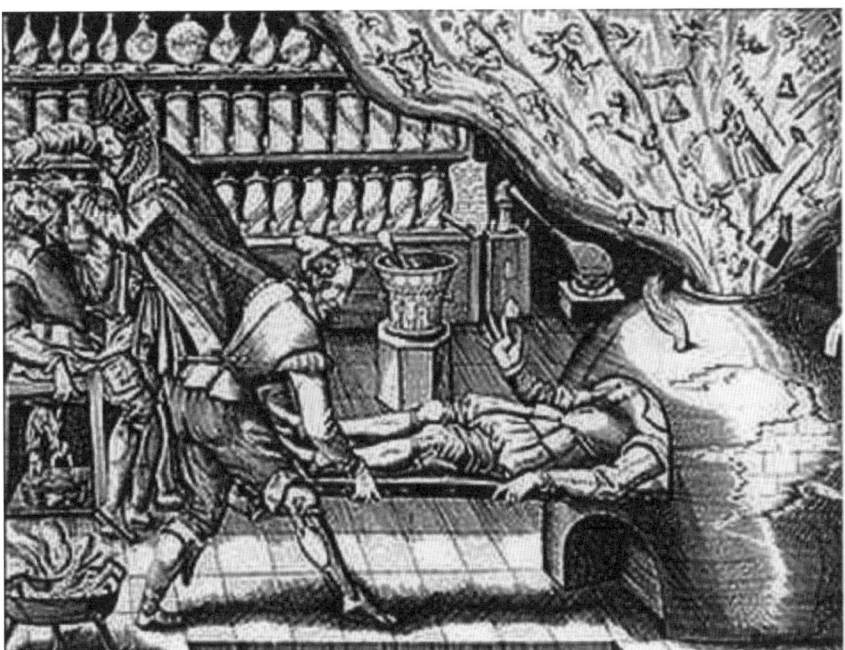

Figure 10.1 Calcination

that aligns with the purpose of the soul. See Figure 10.1 for an interpretation of this.

Calcination can be achieved through a variety of and spiritual, psychological and physical disciplines and by renouncing the material world. By deliberately surrendering our inherent hubris we may burn off our indulgent and excessive nature. This may occur naturally as a result of the humbling process we undergo as we struggle with the trials and tribulations of life.

On a physiological level, the Fire of Calcination can be experienced as an exercise regime or physical discipline that burns off excesses and produces an efficient and finely tuned body.

In the proving the lack of and need for calcinations can be seen in the image produced by the Mini Meditation proving, the fat computer genius living in a world of virtual illusion.

The Tetragrammaton

Last and most important, there is one more reason for my choice of the initial pre-heaven, pre-Hydrogen soul permutation.

This sequence represents an exact replica of Tetragrammaton, the four-letter, holy name of God as written in Hebrew letters from right to left. According to Jewish tradition this name should not be spoken aloud.[i]

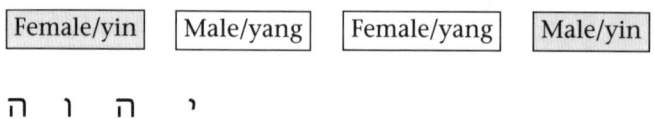

| Female/yin | Male/yang | Female/yang | Male/yin |

ה   ו   ה   י

He who understands will understand.[ii]

References

1   Vital C. Four Aspects of the Emanated. Kabbalah Online, Chabad.org website. Available online at: http://tinyurl.com/7cbhvw4
2   Ezekiel 1:4 Available online at New American Bible Website: http://tinyurl.com/7bn2gym
3   See Alchemy Lab website. Available online at: http://tinyurl.com/6ue8dvc

---

[i] For more on this subject and for correct pronunciation of the tetragrammaton see: Leet L. *The Secret Doctrines of the Kabbalah.* Rochester VT: Inner Traditions International; 1999.

[ii] For a further explanation readers are invited to access the website www.dynamis.edu

11

DIMENSIONS

In our apparent, mundane existence we live in a three-dimensional world composed of lines lying along three directions, up-down, east-west and north-south. It is essential to differentiate between direction (axis) and dimensions. The three directions are height, width and length. The first three dimensions are line, surface and cube. It makes no essential difference what axis each of the three lines lie on, it is the combination of one two or three lines at 90° to each other that forms the three dimensions. Today it is understood that there of many more dimension. Scientists talk in terms of seven, ten and eleven dimensions, which will be discussed later in this series.

During my exploration of the noble gases, I came to understand that each of the periods with its noble gas heralds a new dimension in the space-time continuum. This begins with the singularity of the pre-hydrogen state in which all dimensions are compressed into one. Helium unfolds the first dimension: a line. This line may be placed along length, width or depth; it is just a matter of orientation in space. At a first examination it seems that Helium's direction of line is up-down, with many references to high places, floating, mountains, descending or viewing the world from above. Note however that the axis of the line can change according to the point of view we choose; we may view the Helium line as vertical, running from up down, or as horizontal and splitting the up-down axis. For this discussion I have chosen the first point of view. Changing the axis will lead to some different perceptions, but Helium's confinement to a line remains the same. I will develop this theme further in Neon.

Thus the first period describes the evolution from the non-dimensional, infinitesimal dot of pre-hydrogen to the first dimension of the line. Let us review this process.

The universe supposedly began with a singularity. Physicists say that nothing existed before this singularity and they are right, nothing did exist. We can call this 'dimension zero'. Modern-day physicists do not have the

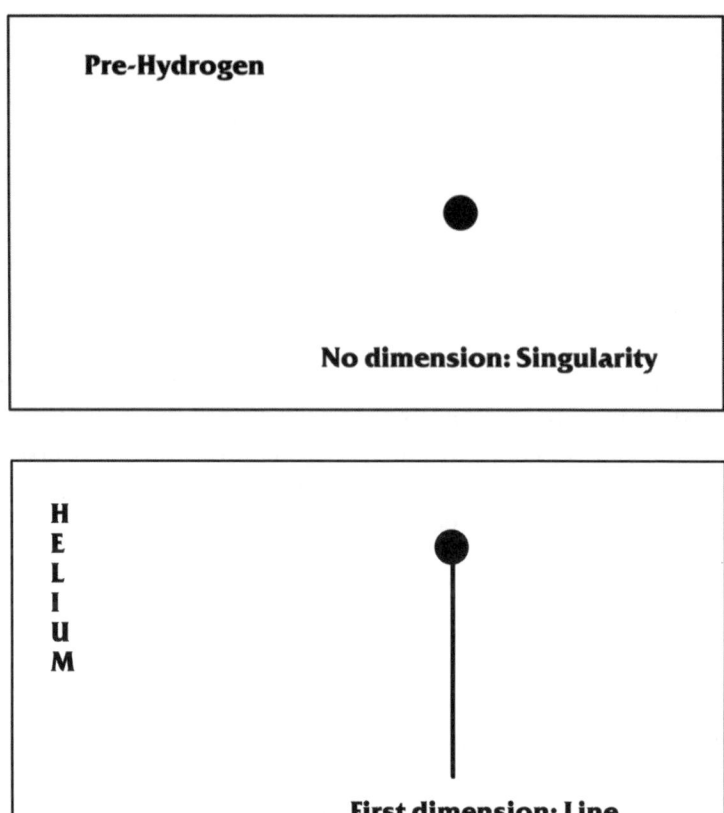

Figure 11.1 *From Hydrogen to Helium: moving into the first dimension*

ability to define this dimension, and so it remains in the realm of poets and priests.

The universe is created by the contraction of no-thing, which consequently leaves some-thing. The something is compressed into a singularity, which has difficulty expanding. This challenge is solved by the Big Bang. The singularity is scattered in all directions, creating unbounded space, which is reflected in the Hydrogen remedy picture. Hydrogen's pathology includes the inability to focus or realise boundaries. This difficulty is solved when hydrogen fuses into helium, creating light. At this stage light travels in a straight line. Thus the Helium solution to Hydrogen's lack of boundaries is to contract into one dimension, a line. This line is vertical, and each Helium soul represents one possible line among the many vertical lines of all the souls. Helium learns how to descend and ascend along this line. Its choice is simple: Either to float above or descend down into the vertex; up or down, spirit or earth, true or false, pure or impure (see Figure 11.1).

The Helium soul is a prisoner of its narrow linear confines, hence the obsessive-compulsive nature of this remedy. While Helium at its high point is an extremely spiritual and free remedy, this view point presents the polarity of a one-dimensional spirituality, with no depth of emotion or human interest. There is much reference to self and spirit and little to 'the other'. If we meet Helium further down the line it depicts a one-sided depravity, with no breadth of morality and no consideration of fellow humans (see the Mini Meditation proving in Chapter 6). I have found that some Helium cases present as one sided and repetitive, and though they touch on spiritual matters, they are confined to one line of thought.

Helium's pathology is a refusal to flex, to move out of its linear existence. For this it will need an extra direction: width. This extra direction will unfurl alongside the second period. To develop this new aspect of existence, the following elements will have to expand into the subtle shades of human existence. This can only be achieved by leaning forward into width and combining both lines to form the second dimension of surface, or line squared. The subsequent elements of Lithium to Neon will learn how to s-t-r-e-t-c-h. Lithium will have to be lithe.

Dark feeling coming down on me. Like a **shadow sinking down from above and behind.** Strong desire to kneel down by the bed, **stretch out** my upper body on the bed and pray. I want to be **carried away, out of this dimension and into another one.** I feel **trapped** inside this confused **head**, which is aching. I wish I could **curl up** in bed and sleep for years – to get away.

Each dimension creates the susceptibility for the next one. By confining itself to a line Helium's movement is constricted to a narrow axis, up and down. By splitting the world in two Helium's line creates a susceptibility for the next dimension. As we descend into the next period this new dimension will develop, creating further possibilities in our world (see Figure 11.2).

At this point I highly recommend watching a short movie clip available online at http://tinyurl.com/ydzsau. This animation illustrates the concepts presented in chapter one of the book *Imagining the Tenth Dimension* by Rob Bryanton.[1]

No matter which dimension we exist in, the next dimension creates a degree of freedom we could not achieve within the current one. These further dimensions seem inconceivable to us from our lesser, more limited perception (much like a sceptic trying to understand homeopathy!). When we do expand into the next dimension, the previous one will inevitably seem superficial and inadequate. This is an important concept, the logic of

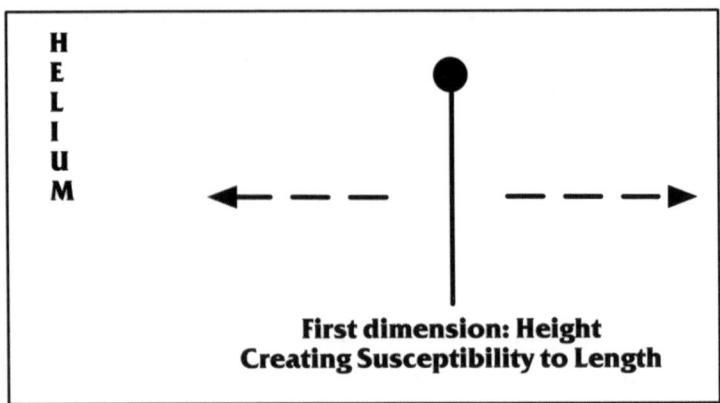

Figure 11.2 *Helium's vertical line results in an up-down split, creating susceptibility to width*

which will continue throughout this series. The question is: What price do we pay for the freedom of new dimensions? Here we must bear in mind the polarity of the great freedom of the soul constricting into a confined material existence, and its desperate attempt to regain that freedom in the world.

In his book *Flatland: A Romance of Many Dimensions* Edwin Abbot describes the reality of a one dimensional world,

> His subjects ... were all alike confined in motion and eyesight to that single Straight Line, which was their World. It need scarcely be added that the whole of their horizon was limited to a Point; nor could anyone ever see anything but a Point.[2]

From Helium's point of view this point corresponds to the higher purpose of it's existence.

A song of great Dimensions

No-thing was every-where
No-thing was every-time.
No-thing was bored.
No-thing decided to pack up its no-things
And go no-where else
But it left some-thing;
A dot

.

Dot was every-thing
Everything was dot.
Dot looked around.
There was no-thing to be seen
Dot tried to move up.
Dot tried to move sideways.
Dot tried to move forward.
It could not It was dot.
Man, this was frustrating
Dot could not take this for much longer.
Dot got all en-tangled with itself
The pressure was building, fast
Dot was getting mad, real mad
Dot was about to expl-!

Bang

Dot was free!
It was heaven, it was bliss
One-thing it was not;
Dot became a No-Dot.

Dot expanded
Up, down, back, forward, sideways,
For a million billion whatevers
Dot pushed its own envelope
Expanding into the No-Nothing
which remained
After No-thing split.

Now No-Dot was Not-Now
And No-Dot was Not-Here
No-Dot had moved somewhere
Between then and there

It rolled and expanded
At incredible pace
Till Not-Now became time
And Not-Here became space

But No-dot was scattered
Battered and shattered
Finding direction
Was all that now mattered

No-Dot was lost
And it looked all around,
No-One to be seen
Not even a sound
It longed for direction
A place to call home
And it wished that no-thing
Would pick up the phone

It wished that no-thing
Would drop it a line
Just then No-thing called
I hope all is fine?

Here is your line
It's called 'I-me-mine'
Please confine to this line
That leads from up down.

A line? That was fine
I will slide down this line
That extends from mid-heaven
Into some-body's spine

In a golden shrine
On top of cloud nine
Line waited its turn
Line bided its time

Photons forged atoms
Helium fused sun
Light banished dark
End of day one

But Line became fixed
Compulsive, Obsessive
Line would not bend
This got quite excessive

Dirty or clean
False or be true
There was really no way
To bridge between two

To be continued . . .

References

1   Bryanton R. *Imagining the Tenth Dimension: A New Way of Thinking About Time and Space*. Bloomington IN: Trafford Publishing; 2006.

2   Abbott EA. *Flatland: A Romance of Many Dimensions. 1884.* Amazon CreateSpace International Publishing Platform; 2013. Available online at: http://tinyurl.com/68km5t

12

PERIOD I SYNTHESIS

I hereby conclude my exploration of Helium.

By perceiving Helium, we perceive Hydrogen. Because it has separated from the oneness of God, Hydrogen must emulate another form of the one: the individual soul. It achieves this by fusing into Helium.

One to one: From God's oneness to the Helium one soul, the first period is complete. Each noble gas is an answer to a question posed by the preceding period, yet every noble gas poses its own question to the following period. While we long to return to what came before, we are forced to move forward and find new solutions.

The periodic table of our evolution is a one-way street. Our true home lies behind us and we yearn for it, yet we are doomed to travel down this road seeking temporary accommodation. A policeman with a revolving laser guards the way back. There is only one way to reverse direction and travel back to the source, and that is by means of a mirror; the law of similars in all its manifestations.

Going the opposite way, it was as if I was in another world. Everyone was appearing so diverse and all men were appearing as one man.

The following synthesis summarises the evolution from pre-Hydrogen to Helium:

Pre-Hydrogen: God is one, everywhere.

God's question: How will you receive?

Solution: God withdraws his oneness. Void leads to singularity leads to Hydrogen.

Hydrogen's pathology: Collective soul fragments. Yearning to return to God.

Hydrogen's question: Where is the one?

Solution: Delusion I am one, a line. Helium.

Helium pathology: Remain in the line. Reluctance to lean forward or split. Yearning to return to the collective soul.

Helium's question: How will I get out of this line?

Solution: Lean and divide. Second period and Neon.

Summary pre-Hydrogen to Helium: From 'God is one' to 'I am one'.

Dimensions: From pre-Hydrogen no-thing to a singular dot, through Hydrogen's unbounded expansion into a Helium line splitting creation into the world above and the world below.

One thing will become clear as we journey through the nobles. While the usual progress of human evolution is along the horizontal line of periods, there is also a direct vertical path running between the nobles, a ladder where one can ascend and descend without the pain and pleasure of the lesser elements. I have found in practice that the noble gases may follow each other well. There is also an overlap between their provings: Helium runs into Neon, Neon to Helium and Argon.

Helium, the individual soul, is the bridge between the first period's universal soul and the subsequent second period. Once the soul incarnates it will need a body. This will be supplied by carbon, oxygen and nitrogen, which form organic life and lends material structure. The body will need water, the union of hydrogen and oxygen and the ultimate bond between the first and second period, soul and body. Yet this water molecule, containing ten protons and ten electrons, is just an emulation of Neon, which has the same number of particles. The whole second period will be longing to go back to Helium, but striving towards Neon.

We will meet at Neon. Don't look back.

Proving symptoms related to Helium MM

Here follows a small yet significant selection of symptoms arranged according to the Helium MM sequence. Some have been abbreviated or grammatically amended for greater clarification, without however altering the original meaning in any way. Please refer to the full proving for a complete list of symptoms.[i]

One sex

I woke and heard someone shout "Dad" and I responded as if they had shouted "Mum". I felt I was both or either.

Sensation as if I don't exist. I felt as if I had a man inside of me in my head and genitally, filled in every way by a man.

Like the yew we come in one sex, unlike angels, so we need to connect with another.

Light-like spirit permeates, pervades all. No need for rights or rituals, veiling in the full glory of spirit. Reverse impressions, my thoughts are blocking the spontaneity, so I withdraw and feel safer. This description was hermetic in an esoteric sense, and also in the sense of an airtight closure by fusion. I was not distracted as a hermaphrodite.

One eye

In my inner vision I kept seeing the eye of Horus. With that image came the thought that a peacock heals in the same way as an emerald.

I was told from the people with one eye. It felt like I was from the people with one eye. The giving was from the people with one eye.

---

[i] A full copy of the proving is available at www.dynamis.edu

From very early times in Egypt, the sun and the moon were regarded as the eyes of the great falcon god Horus. The two eyes eventually became differentiated, with the left eye (the 'eye of Horus') often being regarded as the symbol of the moon and the right eye (the 'eye of Re') being that of the sun. One of the best-known myths concerning the moon relates its cycle to the battle between Horus and Seth. During this famous battle over the inheritance of Osiris, Seth steals the (left) eye of Horus, damages it and divides it into six parts. Thoth (with the help of the other gods) later restores it 'with his fingers' or by spitting on it.

Four in one

The whole issue of destiny. Maybe we are squatters finding our double in another body? I have a sensation that I am looking out of another person's eyes, with three other people.

Dream of being high up in the mountains with a lot of snow. Three cows are coming up the hillside.

Dreamt about four men coming into my life. They were all very different from each other. I woke up with a feeling that a man is coming into my life, all of the four could suit me, not just 'the one'.

The woman had two partners and this was her fourth child but who was the father?

I was waiting for someone to say "I know you", but also pretending I didn't exist – those were the two sides.

I didn't want to use the word 'you', I wanted to add another vowel to it.

I went off and saw a man crouched, and I ran east towards the man who was in front. I then saw a woman who would help, she stood in the north.

I was hoping there would be peace in Hebron.

Double sun

I didn't know whether it was morning or afternoon. I had no concept because it was all light. When I opened my eyes I saw the moon as if it were a second sun and the second sun rose in the east. It was the queen reflecting the brilliance of the king.

The moon, which is archetypical female energy, is as brilliant as the sun. Female energy exposed in all its glory.

I had a thought on waking: The queen is not dead, she's just not always seen due to the brilliance of the king.

Dream: Perfect sun in the day and stars visible in the night, both were bright.

In my inner vision I could see buffalo returning, and a rainbow around the sun which is called Sundog. It felt they were both raising hope in the world. The rainbow around the sun felt that truth shattered the bonds of separation.

Double male

No division, night was as bright as day.

The wand (penis) is double-ended, but one end is circumcised and the other is not.

Circumcision, for what reason? Thoughts on circumcision.

Dream there were two Aryan men, both with large genitalia.

Sensation in my right wrist that it was the same as the other side. Was it left as well? Or inside out?

$2^5 = 32$

In my inner vision I kept seeing griffins. It was about the strength of a lion and the vision of an eagle. This inner vision was all about the vision of an eagle and the heart of a lion – the griffin.

Penetrating wands

Double-ended light

Expanding brilliance

Eternal sun.

Hidden female

The great ambition of women is to inspire love – about double divine twins.

Double withdrawal. Do I perceive the opposite all the time?

I was talking to two older girls in a young school.

They needed partners?

Only fully loving if giving and receiving.

Seeing the invisible in the visible, and the indivisible in the one.

It was dark, I used a long exposure. I wondered whether it would be seen on film because it was so underexposed.

I thought and felt transparent and beautiful inside.

Queen of the heavens with her train of stars.

Eternally expectant, waiting for her king

to be penetrated by the light.

Clear, dark icy night,

warmed and softened in the embrace, with the formation of light, impregnated with stars.

Night in her reflected glory
drawing back her cloak.
Revealing the stars,
guiding us home.
Solstice of darkness
bearing the light.
Receptive is your womb
for receiving the light.
Vessel growing,
in the watery darkness we float.
Hidden for a while
before revealing our gift.
Receiving joyously
so we too may give
All returns to the One.
Banished from home,
night banishes the day.
Night envelops the day.
Night cloaks the day.
Day penetrates with light the night.

Banished so vanish
Out of the darkness light was born, before the flood of human emotion. Yet receptive still, protected, nourished, cradled in the womb. Without cares, within peace. One with our mother, the only movement the spirit. Like the wind over the still, dark waters. Connecting us to life. One two, one two.

Restoring the light to unity. Impregnated darkness, vessels of light. Eternally expectant for the second coming.

Invisible

I pretend I don't exist.

After I didn't exist, I had the delusion I was invisible to others but not invisible to myself.

Delusion of being invisible. Perhaps not making contact and feeling responsible for others' pain.

Seeing the invisible in the visible, and the indivisible in the one.

Fusion

Sudden heat in bursts and in waves, like the heat you get just before an orgasm.

Through the mirror

In the greengrocers I was attracted to one of two young Asian men. I felt the connection via a mirror. There was not the usual feeling of me being unattractive. I thought and felt transparent and beautiful inside. We recognised each other.

If two humans look into a mirror, do they see the same, the opposite or reverse sides? Am I denying soul connections?

The thing about being withdrawn, do people just mirror us? We (humans) certainly don't see the same thing.

Felt like no one would want to mirror me. Is our identity formed through the reflection of others? Do we see ourselves as separate from our mothers?

Unsure of imprints from the outside that I could accept as being true. But do we just see how we are mirrored in others?

Complete the web, enter the mirror, dive into watery reflection.

I lost the frustration of not being understood. I had an internal understanding of others. I felt I could see the self in everyone and in their own reflected image.

Crossover

Dream: I dreamt I was looking after twins crossing a road to join one other. Friends were walking, it was nice to meet up, it was like seeing yourself in everyone as if there were no separation. Then I joined many happy people walking in a line crosswise to meet us. I see the self in everyone and in their own reflected image.

I feel like an empty page, a page embossed but not written on, so do I see and do the reverse?

Felt I was waiting for someone to switch the light on. It felt as if someone had turned the dimmer switch down, plus or minus reality.

Sensation in my right wrist that it was the same as the other side. Was it left as well? Or inside out?

Dream: Dream that a girlfriend of mine took a bath and suddenly changed sex. She said, "Look at me, I washed myself too much." She was very relaxed about it and got back into the bath.

In my inner vision, I was stepping up a step with my left foot but the lace of my shoe was caught under my right foot.

Dream: A man was talking to a transvestite in a blue, stripy dress and jacket. Then there was a man with double jaws: a smaller one within the larger one.

I wanted to shake hands with the wrong hand. This lasted all day

Opposites

I wasn't sure if I was experiencing the opposite of everybody else or whether my interpretation was the opposite. I wasn't sure if it was everybody else or me, but I was experiencing the opposite of everybody else.

Experience was of opposites, yet memory of one.

Felt good in a warm bed or cold air – opposites.

Instead of either/or choice, same thing with two different words for it. No choice, just one option.

The blank page seems open to any impression but it also feels like a closed book. Closed but open – opposites.

I don't actually remember having a mother this time around. All these thoughts are fundamental. Do we search for the same or the opposite?

I felt I appeared opposite to how I felt. I felt graceful and light but I appeared clumsy and heavy.

Reverse

Dream: Recognising when people were unwell by the fact they walked backwards.

Dream: On a bus with my mother going in the wrong direction. We both jumped off and I caught up with the number 11 bus, only because they were loading and unloading old folks in wheel chairs. It was not the 101 but the next 11. At the junction I looked down the left fork and the bus was down the right fork. The eleven doesn't go down either road anyway.

No sleep, no leaving the body, no reprieve, ever more inwards, but I felt I needed to persevere and reverse the process.

Dream: Erosion was caused by a friend in a hurry, trying to find a shortcut over black ribbed rock. He went off the path. As we retraced our steps, they gave way. I caught hold of a horizontal bar and pulled myself up. I was upset at the erosion.

I felt a need to act, not just to think. Do I have to imagine it first? I knew I had to make contact, a very passive state. The will felt strong and I felt I could just reverse things and I wouldn't have to withdraw further.

With writing I felt I could start at the bottom of the page and move up.

Sexual connections

I feel different in the way I relate to others. I don't relate in the same way as others relate to others. Others only connect sexually yet not on other levels. Does this lessen their isolation? I don't feel ready for the world yet. I'm unsure what to do next.

Dream: At last I'm reconnected with my lover, the man I saw double of, but it was dark and I recognised his genitals.

We come in one sex unlike angels so we need to connect with another. Sex seems a very gross way of communicating.

Male and female – this is how it's done on earth. Until this time you were androgynous, you didn't need sex. Along with this thought I was getting wavelike movements of the involuntary muscles of my vagina (multiple orgasm).

Withdrawn emotionally, so much pain. Close off the outside world and retreat. Or try and reconnect sexually? I want to say the first. Two ways. Rather than go for the opposite option.

Dream: a man was talking to a transvestite in a blue, stripy dress and jacket. Then a man with double jaws, a smaller one within the larger.

In my understanding of this proving symptom, a transvestite represents the stage before sexual differentiation. The stripes indicate the relationship of the four entities at this stage.

Genitalia

Dream: I dreamt there were two Aryan men, both with large genitalia.

Circumcision, for what reason?

In my inner vision I was handed a rattle, the body of which was a turtle and the handle was the foreleg of a deer. The handle turned into a penis as I held it and as I handled it I was called 'shining one'. I was told this was a gentle connection with the earth. I knew it was for me and I was shocked by knowing. More wands, I was holding a wand very gently and it became an erect penis.

Dream: I was hugged by a man and my face was level with his crotch (I don't know if I was small or he was big). I felt sad. He said, "Don't be upset", he would find me a man, and then he said, "You blew it".

Womb exchange

Starting two things at once. Where am I? Am I in the right bed or womb? Not sure if I'm in the right womb, is this what I really need ? Fulfilling destiny, second thoughts, it's not doubting, it's second thoughts.

Dream: I dreamt that I was going to give birth to another woman's baby. But it wasn't clear: Was it me who was pregnant and me that was going to give her the baby after the birth? Or was it her that was pregnant and me that was going to have the baby? If I was pregnant, had there been a semen implantation? I was very puzzled by all this in the dream.

Dream: I dreamt my neighbour (in reality) had just had a baby with my girlfriend (she is pregnant). She didn't realise that this baby was already born, and she was still pregnant with another man's child.

Division

I felt only half here, yet functioning very well. I felt clear, efficient, light and calm, as if I had left my other half in a dream. Each half felt complete. Each half was very complete as a whole but it was half.

Dream: I dreamt the coach was in two halves. I was on a single seat on the bus.

I felt the world was not seen as pure enough. I believe none of what I hear and only half of what I see.

Dream: A whole strip of stamps one below the other and the bottom row was ripped off.

As if I was waiting for someone to say "I know you", but also pretending I didn't exist – those were the two sides.

Dream: I dreamt that I was on a plane with no clothes on. I was very happy and I arrived in London dancing. I was on my own as 'I needed to be with light blue'. The dancing was all like this ((()))))((((()()). Like two sides of a circle, waiting for the other side.

Doubles

I was out and saw the double of somebody. With this came the realisation that I was female and not androgynous, like I had seen the masculine aspect. It felt the division was painful while seeing the double, i.e. I saw somebody who couldn't possibly have been there. It was their double and they were there, but I knew it was impossible. It came together with a deep desire to reconnect.

The great ambition of women is to inspire love – about double divine twins.

Dream of a baby born with diabetes. On waking it felt like it was the greatest gift, and with vision it was a double blessing.

Twins

Image of a hand gently holding a penis. With the words "Will you, won't you, will you, won't you? Join the dance?" I heard a voice say, "You know the steps" = initiation of joyous self discovery. Tefnut and snake. The twins, male and female, the union, it was the symbol of male and female union which could be used throughout life as a polarity. Twins, looking at each other, joined, facing each other, union.

Dream of looking after twins crossing a road to join each other. Friends were walking, it was nice to meet up. It was like seeing yourself in everyone as if there is no separation. Then I joined many happy people walking in a line crosswise to meet us. I see the self in everyone, in their own reflected image.

Always seeing both sides makes action difficult. I felt I was seeing the twin of everything but not seeing the double. It was the twin.

I am travelling on a train and two seats in front of me I see a pair of twins and am fascinated by them. They are young men of around 20. They are sitting with their shoulders touching as though they are joined, but turn to face each other when they speak. Their faces look interested and animated when they speak as though there is a lively energy between them. Their conversation is almost a dance. I have rarely seen two people so interested in each other. They look like two aspects of one person. The thought comes to me that this remedy is about moving from the one to the two, close enough still to feel connected but with enough distance to see the beloved.

Diversity

Going in the opposite direction, it was as if I was in another world, everyone appeared so diverse and then all men appeared as one man.

It feels like I am stepping from the oneness to the twoness.

Soul DNA

First images: That this remedy is about re-grouping into a group with people you really want to be with and who are really on the same path as you.

Image of spiralling downwards through lilacs and mauves.

I have an image of a school sports team and choosing the side you want to be on, then changing sides at the last minute as you realise you would in fact rather be on the other team.

A spiral maze. The spiral of the self and the search for self, symbolising the wandering of the soul circling inward and outward, seeking nourishment and experience from the outside and from within itself to finally achieve its goal of enlightenment. Your spiralling dance through life also turns you outward, linking you with others through the group soul or collective unconscious that pervades and encompasses all life. You have a part to play to assist in the spiritual journey of others as they also do in yours.

The ivy puts you in touch with your own inner resources giving you the ability to see through the eyes of the soul beyond the everyday world. The colour associated with the Ogham[i] is sky blue. Retain a vision of the clear blue sky to which you aspire in your mind's eye.

I lost the frustration of not being understood. I had an internal understanding of others. I felt I could see the self in everyone and in their own reflected image.

I wasn't sure if I was experiencing the opposite of everybody else or whether my interpretation was opposite. I wasn't sure it was everybody else or me, but I was experiencing the opposite of everybody else.

Dream: Cars that said 10 but it was actually 12.

Dream: A whole strip of stamps one below the other and the bottom row was ripped off.

In the greengrocers I was attracted to one of two young Asian men. I felt the connection via a mirror.

Do people just mirror us? Unsure of imprints from the outside to accept as being true, but do we just see how we are mirrored in others?

Separation of side by side. Standing together, of side by side, roots intertwining. Toe to toe, touch of hands.

Dream: On a bus with my mother going in the wrong direction. We both jumped off and I caught up with the number 11 bus only because they were loading and unloading old folks in wheelchairs. It was not the 101 but the next 11. At the junction I looked down the left fork and the bus was down the right fork. The eleven doesn't go down either road anyway.

I felt the only way I could communicate was to lie down beside somebody.

Going in the opposite way, it was as if I were in another world. Everyone was appearing so diverse and then all men were appearing as one man.

---

[i] Ogham is an early medieval alphabet used primarily to write the Old Irish language and occasionally the Brythonic language.

I joined many happy people walking in a line crosswise to meet us. I see the self in everyone, in their own reflected image.

Reflection of the other
Mirror of opposites.
Waiting to be invited
To join the dance.
Creating vessels not vehicles
For easy passage.
Sunbeams (sun beams),
So we dance,
Spiralling together,
Tentatively at first,
Around each other.
Entwining then,
Touching yet,
How can this be?
Spirit soars,
Soul sings,
Together again,
At last,
As first.
In the beginning
There was one
Who became two.
Separated,
In order to multiply,
Returning to the one,
Go forth and multiply.

The dancing was all like this ((())))))((((()())). Like two sides of a circle, waiting for the other side. I looked across and saw a man, unpartnered. He started walking around towards me.

She is playing patience, laying the cards down quickly and deliberately in their sequences, deftly moving them around (is it clock patience?). Her hands are like great graceful spiders, poised and then pouncing. She seems depressed? Irritable? She mutters something about 'males' without looking up from the game. I look at the cards. She is moving all the picture cards. I am very aware of the jacks, queens, kings, all the royals being moved about meaningfully.

Dreams about finding the innate energy pattern of each person in order to help heal them or reactivate their energies.

Epilogue: Helium transferring to Neon

The following are Helium symptoms that either relate to the Neon proving or are shared by it. When the noble gases are aligned, there is a direct connection between them and we can progress directly from one to the next. This has been borne out in the provings, as well as in the relationship of these remedies in clinical practice. I have noticed that the noble gases often follow each other well in clinical practice.

Knocking on the door, didn't go to open it.

Keys broken in locks.

Delusion at night that I could hear the phone ringing or knocking.

Second or fifth day, take us back through timeless state (the angels do all the praising and adoring on the second day and on the fifth day they do all the work) The second day ones were like archangels.

Sensation as if slipping over on ice.

Out in the snow excited by emerald heads of mallards, I felt like a duck on ice.

In my inner vision I could see stars that looked like snow, and snow looking like stars falling very gently. Ameliorated by silence and the purity of snow.

Complete the web, enter the mirror, dive into watery reflection.

In the morning, dawn the opening of a radiant eye. I felt Neon was seeing the eye, but Helium was seeing through the eye.

Yet before the waters of emotion.

Queen of the heavens

Honouring her King.

Leaving the waters of home? We grow towards the light.

White birds.

Inner vision stuff of swans. The swan said you are one of us, fly south and play.

I kept seeing swans in my inner vision.

Inner vision of Pegasus – things with white wings.

I was in some Japanese-inspired surroundings. An egg-shaped pond with ice-cold water, and a thin layer of ice on top. I didn't know if it was muddy or full of plants, fishes, other creatures, or anything dangerous. I undressed completely and jumped in after a short hesitation. The others around thought it was a great, impressive, respectful thing to do. My body broke the ice as I jumped into the pool. The water was ice-cold but clear. I went all the way to the bottom and then rose slowly upwards. The sun was shining through the water making all the bubbles glitter. I had to take a deep breath while still under water and found that I could breathe in the water. When I broke through the top it was like going through a membrane. I rose from the pond feeling like a new person, a cleaned person, actually more 'me' than ever. I was in contact with all of myself, and felt very whole. It felt like an initiation, and I was met with deep respect afterwards. Right next to the Japanese garden was a farm with a square swimming pool like an American pool. People were swimming, screaming, shouting, laughing, acting rather hysterical, thinking they were having a great time. Some of them had been drinking. It all seemed very superficial compared to the quietness and spirituality right next door. But I felt I was a part of them too – or they were a part of me. I knew what I wanted, how I preferred to be and which part of me I wanted to live. When undressing to go into the pond I felt very shy and naked; on rising from the pond the nakedness was in a way spiritual, with no shyness.

Miscellaneous symptoms of special interest.

The following symptoms do not fit into any one particular category, yet they contain many images and concepts that illuminate Helium and the world beyond.

Another time than ours, it stretched across different centuries. An old kingdom, a lot of people, parties, wars and violence. I was married to the king, but he never touched me. Other men took me, but it didn't concern me. I felt at a distance, like an observer. I felt a stranger, so bad things didn't hurt me. A bear hunter came, he fascinated me, he took me and I became pregnant. I felt very connected to him. He was wearing a thick, bearskin coat. He came from the outside, was a stranger, kind of timeless. He belonged to any time, but he was also very present in the actual time at the moment. He could fit into any time, but was himself whatever time he moved in and he was always respected as himself.

Thoughts and images of giants. Giants riding on a horse-drawn cart, and also images of seeds, grain and field mice. We all go to the place where Tibetan monks are creating a sand mandala. The countryside looks exactly as I had envisaged it. It was a pleasant, relaxing and soothing experience. The mandala was very beautiful and the colours were bright and clear. It had been created from the centre outwards with infinite patience until it filled the whole square. One of the most fascinating things to watch was how the monks dealt with any mistakes. The misplaced grains of sand were gently moved to the right place, carefully and with no sense of hurry or frustration. There was a great sense of patient acceptance and a sureness of purpose.

During meditation I see myself and everyone, everything with which I am in relationship in a coloured, spinning sphere. I feel my heart being opened to receive love. It feels like an attunement to love. Afterwards I have the thought that the heart needs to be opened twice, once to give love and once to receive love. I have never felt like this before.

I had another night of deeply comforting sleep. It is as if I go to another place when I sleep, somewhere in nature like a moss-lined hollow or cave. There is a sense of deep, deep softness and dryness and a powdery fragrance. The colours I sense are deep blue, indigo and dark green. There is also a sense of being watched over, attended to, and comforted by figures in robes, maybe nuns or monks.

When things have been difficult I have often said how I wished it were possible to have a letter from God every Monday morning with clear instructions and reassurances. This piece of wood feels like that letter from God.

I feel like I am connected to the truth, to the real world, like I am seeing beyond the illusion.

Absolutely terrifying dream and the feeling stays with me after I wake. It takes nearly all day to shake the feeling of fear even though I am very busy and have no time to dwell on it. I am in a city with friends and family. We are safe here but we all know that members of a religious cult who kidnap people live close by. I am walking down a familiar street when I feel a hand on my arm and I know it is one of them. My friends have disappeared. Immediately I know I have to keep my nerve, pretend I am going along with them and not show fear. The person who has captured me is a man wearing shiny clothes. All the cult members wear clothes made from this fabric and sometimes robes. We smile and chat. He tells me how much I will enjoy working with his friends then takes me into a big building to meet the other cult members. Everyone is busy working. I don't understand what they are doing but pretend to be interested. All the time I feel so terrified that I can hardly breathe, all the time I am making plans in my head to escape, looking for an opportunity to get away. I tell myself to keep my nerve all the time. I smile and smile and pretend I am going along with it. Then I am taken to meet the man I'll be working with. He is very old and thin, wears robes and looks quite mad. He is holding on tightly to a woman who has her back to me and he tells me how well the three of us will work together. Then I see he is holding her so she cannot turn round and see me but I catch a glimpse of her profile and see she is wearing a black band to cover her eyes. My blood runs cold because I know for sure that this man has cut her eyes out. The man and I smile and smile at each other. We each know the other is bluffing but I am going to win this game.

Shortly afterwards I just walk out of the building towards the streets that I feel safe in. Several cult members follow me and hold my hand or arm. I have to keep my nerve, it is a bluffing game. I say that I am just going to walk to this corner and oh, there is an interesting shop over there in the next street and gradually I lose them as they cannot hold me. Then I am free of them. I woke with a gasp and my heart was beating fast. The dream is about staying with what you absolutely know to be the truth no matter how sinister your surroundings or what horrors people conjure up.

Dream: About the Divine Masculine and how it was the right time for it to be brought down more fully into physical manifestation. I was told that this process had begun with George Harrison's death, but there was lots of work to be done on it this year. I was told that during the next women's group at Beltane we should honour the Divine Masculine and invite the energy in as though we were goddesses choosing the Year King. I heard, "It is the Goddess that makes the God, the woman that makes the man." I was told the precise way to go about it, that we should begin by each saying what qualities we thought were Divine Masculine qualities and then invite that divine man in. I was told that if we did this in one particular way we would each conjure up a man that we would meet, but that was not the purpose and it would all end in tears anyway. Our purpose was a more advanced and subtle magic, to bring down the Divine Masculine energy.

Dream: I woke from a dream about love and duality, the power of the two. The dream images were vague but the story had been about rescuing someone through love. The experience of doing it was the most important thing. It was as though I was being taught how to do it. I had some words of a song about love in my head and movements that went with the words. I sang it in my head over and over again and felt myself dissolving into love.

All day I felt in a languorous mood. I looked the word up in the diction-ary. It means softest and most tender mood. All day I felt I could do or change anything in the whole world by aligning myself to that love and bringing it into any and every situation in life. I felt very purposeful. I did not want to speak very much. All day I have felt connected to love and even the air feels soft and easy to breathe. It feels like I am stepping from the oneness to the twoness. At the end of the day my husband told me he thought I could have changed the whole world that day. He said I was very magical.

Dream of packing to go back home. Skateboarding, then snowboarding down through a car park and roads towards the bus stop. Going to the bus stop to catch the train with many others. In a hotel, a little girl ran off and I went to find her. She and I spotted my ex-husband perched in a tree that was hanging over the water, taking photos of the water or something in the water. I took a photo of him and he spotted us. It was dark, I used a long exposure. I wondered whether it would not be seen on film because it was so underexposed.

Dream: Before departing for Israel I was running like the wind and I let my hair free. As I ran like the wind, I sank into shallow water. I had a flat stomach. I swam, avoiding drowned cars, and swam against the current to reach a sand bank where I was going to body surf. I was packing to go to Israel and meeting up with him to go to the desert, it felt like things were very unfinished and needed to be completed.

INDEX

Entries associated with the case studies are shown with **bold** page numbers. Page numbers in *italics* show figures and diagrams